Elements of culture and mental health: critical questions for clinicians

Edited by Kamaldeep Bhui

RCPsych Publications

© The Royal College of Psychiatrists 2013

RCPsych Publications is an imprint of the Royal College of Psychiatrists,
17 Belgrave Square, London SW1X 8PG
http://www.rcpsych.ac.uk

British Library Cataloguing-in-Publication Data.
A catalogue record for this book is available from the British Library.
ISBN 978 1 908020 49 9

Distributed in North America by Publishers Storage and Shipping Company.

The views presented in this book do not necessarily reflect those of the Royal College of
Psychiatrists, and the publishers are not responsible for any error of omission or fact.

The Royal College of Psychiatrists is a charity registered in England and Wales (228636)
and in Scotland (SC038369).

Printed by Bell & Bain Limited, Glasgow, UK.

Contents

List of contributors

Imran Ali Consultant Psychiatrist, Greater Manchester West NHS Foundation Trust, Manchester, and Member of the Spiritual Care Committee, NHS Greater Glasgow and Clyde, UK

Jorge Atala-Delgado Psychologist and Anthropologist, Anahuac and Chapultepec University, Mexico City, Mexico

Kamaldeep Bhui Professor of Cultural Psychiatry and Epidemiology, Barts and the London School of Medicine and Dentistry, Queen Mary, University of London, and Honorary Consultant Psychiatrist, East London NHS Foundation Trust, London, UK

Francisco Collazos Associate Professor of Psychiatry, Universitat Autònoma de Barcelona, and Servei de Psiquiatriá, Hospital Universitari, Vall d'Hebron, Barcelona, Spain

Francisco José Eiroa-Orosa Psychologist, Servei de Psiquiatriá, Hospital Universitari, Vall d'Hebron, CIBERSAM, and Universitat Autònoma de Barcelona, Spain

Peter Ferns Training Consultant and Social Worker, Thornton Heath, UK

Maria José Fernandez-Gomez Psychologist, Servei de Psiquiatriá, Hospital Universitari, Vall d'Hebron, CIBERSAM, and Universitat Autònoma de Barcelona, Spain

Suman Fernando Honorary Professor, Faculty of Social Sciences and Humanities, London Metropolitan University, London, UK

Marcos González Adjunct Psychiatrist, Centre de Salut Mental d'Adults d'Horta, Barcelona, Spain

David Kingdon Professor of Mental Health Care Delivery, University of Southampton, Southampton, UK

Farooq Naeem Consultant Psychiatrist, Sevenacres, St Mary's Hospital, Newport, Isle of Wight, UK

Adil Qureshi Psychologist, Servei de Psiquiatriá, Hospital Universitari Vall d'Hebron, Barcelona, Spain

Shanaya Rathod Consultant Psychiatrist and Clinical Service Director, Southern Health NHS Foundation Trust, Southampton, UK

Hilda-Wara Revollo Psychologist, Servei de Psiquiatriá, Hospital Universitari Vall d'Hebron, and Doctoral Candidate, Universitat Autònoma de Barcelona, Spain

Faisil Sethi Consultant in Psychiatric Intensive Care, Maudsley Hospital, South London and Maudsley NHS Foundation Trust, London, UK

Rachel Tribe Professor of Applied Psychology, School of Psychology, University of East London, London, UK

Premila Trivedi Mental Health Service User, Trainer and Advisor, Thornton Heath, UK

Desire and commitment: essential ingredients to learning about culture and mental illness

Kamaldeep Bhui

The influence of a person's cultural background includes childhood experiences of parenting, rituals and routines informed by religions, and cultural beliefs about the world and the way it works, about supernatural forces and the Gods, and about relationships and emotions. Some people recognise early on in life that their skin colour or their physical appearance, their clothing or their religion's adornments attract curiosity and attention. Sometimes this is hostile, sometimes inquisitive but dismissive, and sometimes it comes of genuine interest to learn about another way of seeing the world.

For Black and minority ethnic groups, discrimination and stigma compound inequalities of the experience and outcome of mental illness. Inequalities arise through interactions between culture/ethnicity and many other factors, such as gender, age and sexuality, not to mention migration experiences, conflict in the country of origin, hostility in the country of arrival, and poverty and social adversity. Such influences exist within and outside formal healthcare systems. Health practitioners are increasingly interested in preventive psychiatry or public mental health, a process of understanding and removing social and environmental determinants of illness, alongside providing health promotion to boost people's capacity to care for themselves and their families.

Cultural practices are known to assist in coping with distress and with interpersonal problems, but they can sometimes also be the source of role conflict and distress within families. The role of cultural beliefs, attitudes and practices is well established in the experience, expression and management of mental distress. Some manage distress through what we might call the lay referral system, which involves the community, the family and local social systems, including religion and spiritual leaders; others enter sanctioned systems of healthcare provision through the self-referral of formal help-seeking.

These cultural influences can pose a challenge for mental health professionals. Mental health professionals work across the interface of many clinical, practical and academic disciplines. Their task is to assess, formulate, diagnose and intervene effectively using the evidence base, and to ensure that interventions are culturally appropriate, acceptable and also ethical – for example, the principles of social justice must be upheld, and human rights and dignity protected. The way they respond to this challenge is mixed. Some feel disempowered by allegations of poor care made by service users, some feel that their professional training is sufficient, and some that universal principles of treating all in the same way apply, regardless of the research evidence showing that this is not always helpful. Indeed, aspirations to provide personal care and person-centred care require such universal interventions to be adapted to take account of each service user's preferences. Some practitioners respond to the need to improve practice by seeking out support workers, or trying to show workforce representation from the communities which are served. But in this they again may overlook the fact that ways of seeing and treating mental distress are culturally influenced, and that cultures influence professional practice as well as lay perspectives; thus, irrespective of their cultural backgrounds, professionals are trained in similar ways and have to work to the same ethical and professional guidelines, which may not service culturally diverse populations well.

Where the research evidence is lacking, there is often scope for stereotyping or for speculative interventions or, indeed, for complacency and professional narcissism, to subvert efforts to tackle ethnic and cultural disparities. Some like to see cultural psychiatry and related disciplines as only serving the interests of ethnic and visible minorities, rather than as part of the fabric of psychiatric practice, of relevance to all service users: do we not all have a culture? Clearly, where the culture of the service user and the professional differs, there is scope for miscommunication, misunderstandings, assumptions and oversights; this can apply to all practice, but is particularly heightened and evidenced in the care of culturally diverse populations.

Yet, what is being asked of mental health professionals is very complex: to acknowledge a lack of experience and expertise in a specific area of knowledge and practice, which affects different populations in different ways; to be prepared to work with culturally diverse populations, who may not expect the same sort of treatments or interventions or even assessment processes as the cultural majority. Health literacy, educational experiences, linguistic proficiency and social determinants of illness vary by cultural and ethnic group; so health professionals providing care for culturally diverse populations have a more demanding task, for example, in working through interpreters or understanding non-adherence. In services that are already stretched and are high-risk environments, practice is largely defensive and perhaps even minimises emotional contact with the service user. Asking professionals for more, both personally and professionally, is met with mixed reactions. These range from avoidance, minimisation ('We have people from *x* background working in our team and we don't need more skills or knowledge than that'), to engagement but subversion of the task, to open hostility and claims that politics and healthcare should not mix. What leads to these strong reactions? How can professionals work confidently with people from diverse cultural backgrounds, engage with the emotional and professional demands, and be more creative in improving the quality of care and the take up of services?

This task has attracted a great deal of concerted effort from the Royal College of Psychiatrists, its chief executive, consecutive presidents and Transcultural Special Interest Group, and from international bodies such as the World Psychiatric Association and the World Association of Cultural Psychiatry. Some years ago, discussions of a working group led by Dr Parimala Moodley resulted in changes to the Royal College of Psychiatrists' training curriculum and to the question bank for the College's Membership examination (the MRCPsych). The group agreed that a training manual would be a helpful resource, but at the time the evidence base was rapidly growing and textbooks of cultural psychiatry were becoming increasingly prominent. To assemble everything needed in a training manual, to make it accessible and comprehensive were deemed to be desirable but unrealistic objectives. An essential component of cultural competence is the inherent recognition of the need to improve care, coupled with the desire to do so. My experience is that this is where most practitioners have difficulty: they have to become interested and motivated in this subject, as opposed to feeling persecuted, avoidant or even oppositional. Placing emphasis on education rather than personal development or on technical knowledge rather than emotional engagement with patients can be counterproductive, and may become an obstacle to improving quality. Some practitioners still ask, what do we need to do and how do we do it? These sentiments convey powerlessness and a sense of bewilderment.

This short volume, developed by service users, practitioners, teachers and researchers, aims to address this dilemma. Its objective is to offer readers a concise, thought-provoking, engaging and creative set of essays about clinical scenarios that are central to improving the quality of care for culturally diverse populations. The scenarios are common, and the essays set out beautifully, examining some of the obstacles to improving quality as well as ways in which dilemmas facing the clinician can present, and how they might be overcome.

The primary purpose of this book is to encourage practitioners to become curious and think about the issues in detail, and to motivate them to seek out further information, learning and experiences. The book can be used to support individual and group professional development. Each chapter includes a set of references, and some chapters also list useful websites and reference materials, and helpful organisations. There are many sources of support. For example, in the UK several practice groups meet regularly, and the College's Transcultural Special Interest Group regularly runs conference and learning events. The World Association of

Cultural Psychiatry offers an open-access online journal (*World Cultural Psychiatry Research Review*) and events and discussion forums. Several other journals are devoted to this subject (for example, *Transcultural Psychiatry* and *International Journal of Culture and Mental Health*). The Transcultural Section of the World Psychiatric Association also runs events, often in collaboration with the World Association of Cultural Psychiatry. Affiliated membership organisations from around the world have demonstrated the level of interest in this subject. There are centres of excellence in universities running MSc and MA courses, for example at McGill University in Montreal and at Queen Mary, University of London. There are e-learning resources such as the Royal College of Psychiatrists' CPD online modules (www.psychiatrycpd.co.uk), which make learning any time and any place a reality. However, to proceed to these advanced learning experiences and courses, and to feel comfortable and motivated to attend such meetings, most practitioners need to have some core concepts and thinking tools, which this book provides. Enjoy the learning and the challenges, and please become a leader in the field by helping develop further resources.

CHAPTER 1

Is trauma-focused therapy helpful for survivors of war and conflict?

Rachel Tribe

Few would argue that war and conflict do not affect those involved, either at the time or afterwards. The useful question to consider is: what are their psychological effects and what are the most appropriate paradigms and descriptors to use for these effects that will be both meaningful and useful to survivors wherever they may be living?

People affected by war and conflict often face a whole series of challenges. In addition to dangers to life and limb, there may be loss of family members, loss of financial security and personal safety, loss of property and of livelihood; there may also be existential losses such as hopes and plans for the future. That war can cause psychological distress appears incontrovertible, but whether this is best described within a narrowly individualistic, medicalised psychiatric framework and symbolised by a diagnosis of post-traumatic stress disorder (PTSD), or within a wider framework that accounts for practical and human loss and distress at the individual and community level is contested in the literature (for a full review of this debate see Bracken & Petty, 1998; Summerfield, 1999; Yule, 1999; Rousseau & Measham, 2007).

Concepts of trauma and traumatisation are, of course, broader than just PTSD but this term has been widely and sometimes uncritically used in relation to war and conflict. The word trauma has been used to explain both an event such as war and a reaction to it, perhaps erroneously linking cause and effect in a rather less complicated way than is found in reality. So the language and descriptors have not always been as accurate as they might be, perhaps adding to confusion about ways of working with individuals or communities after the event and sometimes leading to an over-medicalised discourse. Some believe that war and conflict can traumatise entire communities, whereas others believe that very few people actually develop symptoms that would lead to a diagnosis of PTSD (Summerfield, 1999). Bracken (1998) and Summerfield (1999) have noted the difficulties associated with the concept of PTSD, which include the unquestioning use of a Western world view and the imposition of this in what might be viewed as a patronising manner. In addition, 'PTSD' may describe what is actually a normal human response to abnormal events, promoting a label of individual pathology. Time is also an intervening variable, as is the fact that each individual will react differently to war and conflict. Protective factors include the meanings attributed by individuals and communities affected by war and conflict, the support systems available, and resilience at the individual and community level. The paradigms and descriptors used may define what kind of help is offered and to whom.

Collective trauma or war-time spirit?

Somasundaram (2007) developed the notion of collective trauma on the basis of his work during civil wars in Cambodia and Sri Lanka. It describes the situation in which entire communities are affected by conflict and fail to function as successfully as they did before. Every layer of a community can be disturbed. For example, family relationships, peer groups and social structures can become fragmented and altered. Alternatively, a 'war-time spirit' can emerge, when communities feel strengthened and emboldened by a sense of collective engagement, purpose and support. By its very persistence, an ongoing war is different in nature from a one-off incident such as a train crash (McNally, 2010). People living in a war zone may develop ways of coping at the individual and collective level, although these may not always be psychologically healthy (Somasundaram, 2007). Such ways of thinking about conflict and the mind move away from an individualised model and raise for the psychiatrist challenges concerning interventions and help that will maximise recovery of individuals and their communities. In long-running wars and conflicts, young people may have no experience of living in a peaceful society, which poses special challenges for any engagement.

The debate is further complicated by the matter of the appropriateness of applying Western international psychiatric diagnostic categories to people from communities that have their own descriptors and ways of managing distress (which are not necessarily predicated on a psychiatric framework) in terms, for example, of cultural or religious practices (see Chapter 9, this volume). Humanitarian agencies have often (and with the best of intentions) tried to export, from one population to another, methods of working with people and communities who have been through traumatic events. However, these are not always culturally appropriate and they can undermine traditional systems of coping and help. It has been argued that this is a form of neo-colonialism which assumes that Western models are best and treats individuals as passive recipients in need of external help (Summerfield, 1999). The active participation of communities and internally displaced people has often been missing in work with communities and individuals affected by war and conflict (Weerackody & Fernando, 2011). This is at odds with good clinical and community practice and governance and the development of appropriate services or resources.

At the end of 2010, an estimated 43.7 million people worldwide were forcibly displaced by war and civil conflict (Office of the United Nations

High Commissioner for Refugees, 2011). Families may be dispersed and parents can become practically and psychologically unavailable to their children. In its guidance on treating PTSD, the National Institute for Health and Clinical Excellence (NICE) specifically states that 'Being a refugee is not a diagnosis, and refugees may present with any of the psychiatric disorders or none at all' (National Collaborating Centre for Mental Health, 2006: p. 120).

An equal and respectful dialogue between people from different cultures needs to be established, to ensure that an equal partnership is in place and that any mental health help is meaningful, and culturally and resource appropriate. If an intervention is not meaningful or culturally appropriate it is unlikely to be taken up or be viewed as being of benefit to potential users. Services should build on what individuals and communities know about their own survival and coping systems, and strategies based on these are likely to be both more appropriate and more effective (Tribe & de Silva, 1999; Wessells, 1999). The importance of community engagement in improving health in the UK population has been noted by NICE, which has developed specific guidance on the subject (National Institute for Health and Clinical Excellence, 2008). In addition, best practice in health and social care services stresses the role of service user involvement to ensure that services are appropriate and accessible. Although research shows that this is often more an ambition than a reality (Crawford *et al*, 2003), it should still be a goal.

Many UK and international organisations offer information, guidance and support for people affected by war and conflict and for services helping them (Box 1.1). However, as touched on above, international responses to catastrophe can result in aid and personnel being flown in and imposed on the local community. Dawes & Cairns (1998) draw attention to the fact that differential power relations between local and foreign helpers and systems can affect the effectiveness of psychosocial interventions. There are many examples of people from high-income countries imposing models such as trauma counselling on people from other cultures, for whom they are not always appropriate or helpful (Bracken, 1998). The Inter-Agency Standing Committee (IASC) was established in 1992 in response to a United Nations resolution that called for strengthened coordination of humanitarian emergency assistance (United Nations General Assembly, 1991). The resolution identified the IASC as the primary mechanism for facilitating inter-agency decision-making in response to complex emergencies and natural disasters.

Guidelines have been developed by a range of UN and non-UN humanitarian organisations to enable humanitarian actors to plan, establish and coordinate a set of minimum multisectoral responses to protect and improve people's mental health and psychosocial well-being in emergency settings (Inter-Agency Standing Committee, 2007). They propose a model that embeds psychological support within a framework of other measures.

Box 1.1   Organisations offering information, guidance and support

Children and War Foundation
Ensures that knowledge about children can be gathered and used to improve the care of all children affected by war and disaster (www.childrenandwar.org)

Freedom from Torture (Medical Foundation for the Care of Victims of Torture)
Provides information for people working with survivors of torture and organised violence, including how to make a clinical referral and a referral for medico-legal reports (www.freedomfromtorture.org)

International Committee of the Red Cross/Red Crescent
Runs a tracing service for people who have lost contact with family members through a war or on any other grounds (www.icrc.org/familylinks)

International Society for Traumatic Stress Studies
International, interdisciplinary professional organisation that promotes the advancement and exchange of knowledge about traumatic stress (www.istss.org)

Refugee Council
Provides multilingual information for asylum seekers and refugees, news, up-to-date policy and information briefings, guidance for advisors and service providers, specialist country information and a free emailed weekly newsletter about issues relevant to refugees and those working alongside them in the UK (www.refugeecouncil.org.uk)

Refugee Legal Centre
Offers legal advice and representation for asylum seekers and refugees, delivers training and support to those giving advice/representation and seeks to promote the interests of clients individually and through law and public policy. The service is free for those who do not have to pay for legal representation. It also provides advice for detained asylum seekers (www.refugee-legal-centre.org.uk)

United Nations High Commission on Refugees (UNHCR)
Provides press releases and information about refugee situations worldwide, regional overviews and background information as well as statistical and other resources (www.unhcr.org)

World Health Organization (WHO)
The WHO's Humanitarian Health Action states that 'The primary objective in an emergency, whether natural or man-made, is to reduce avoidable loss of life and the burden of disease and disability [...] During crises, humanitarian health partners, led by the Inter-Agency Standing Committee (IASC) Health Cluster under the leadership of WHO will empower humanitarian country teams to better address the health aspects and crises' (http://www.who.int/hac/about/faqs/en/index.html). Its 2001 World Health Report focuses on mental health (www.who.int/whr2001/2001)

The six core principles of action are to:

- ensure human rights and equity
- maximise the participation of the affected population
- do no harm

- build on available resources and capacities
- ensure integrated support systems
- develop multilayered, complementary supports.

Services in the UK

Certain asylum seekers and refugees in the UK may benefit from Tier 3 services that specialise in traumatic stress and use a biomedical and diagnostic model. (The UK Trauma Group lists local resources at www.uktrauma.org.uk/ukservcs.html.) However, for the specific treatment of PTSD, the NICE guidelines recommend cognitive–behavioural therapy (CBT) and eye movement desensitisation and reprocessing (EMDR), but refer to 'barriers to treatment' for refugees and asylum seekers. Consequently, special consideration needs to be given to the requirements of these individuals and to the appropriateness of treatments. One that might usefully deconstruct the phrase 'barriers to treatment' here, as it seems to imply that the asylum seekers are a problem for the treatment, rather than that the treatment might not be the most appropriate for their needs. This is an area of debate in the literature and among professionals.

Other services have developed a more holistic approach, viewing context and culture as organising concepts and regarding the stress of living through war and conflict as extremely challenging but not an experience that leads to a diagnosis of PTSD. Trauma-focused therapy can inadvertently minimise survival skills and resourcefulness and give individuals a diagnostic label that may not be beneficial to their recovery and long-term well-being. This can happen if the treatment is offered indiscriminately and does not account for contextual and cultural factors as well as coping strategies.

Diverse cultures position individuals with psychiatric diagnoses in particular ways. The dilemma, however, is that a psychiatric diagnosis is often a gateway to resources in a system that is often politicised and can be antagonistic to an asylum seeker's needs and even their very presence in the UK. For example, a PTSD diagnosis might be perceived to lend credence to a claim of persecution, thus supporting a request for refugee status under the 1951 UN Convention Relating to the Status of Refugees. This can be highly beneficial to an asylum seeker and may in itself offer significant mental health benefits, as the individual knows that they will not be deported from the UK to their country of origin. Therefore obtaining this diagnosis could be seen as highly functional for the individual. The role of the psychiatrist is therefore a complex one that requires careful consideration and reflection.

References and further reading

Bracken, P. J. (1998) Hidden agendas: deconstructing post traumatic stress disorder. In *Rethinking the Trauma of War* (eds P. J. Bracken & C. Petty), pp. 10–38. Free Association Books.

Bracken, P. J. & Petty, C. (eds) (1998) *Rethinking the Trauma of War*. Free Association Books.

Crawford, M. J., Aldridge T., Bhui, K., *et al* (2003) User involvement in the planning and delivery of mental health services: a cross-sectional survey of service users and providers. *Acta Psychiatrica Scandinavica*, **6**, 410–414.

Dawes, A. & Cairns, E. (1998) The Machel Report: dilemmas of cultural sensitivity and universal rights of children. *Peace and Conflict: Journal of Peace Psychology*, **4**, 335–348.

Inter-Agency Standing Committee (2007) *IASC Guidelines on Mental Health and Psychosocial Support in Emergency Settings*. IASC (http://www.who.int/mental_health/emergencies/guidelines_iasc_mental_health_psychosocial_june_2007.pdf).

McNally, R. (2010) Can we salvage the concept of psychological trauma. *Psychologist*, **5**, 386–389.

National Collaborating Centre for Mental Health (2006) *Post-traumatic Stress Disorder (PTSD): The Management of PTSD in Adults and Children in Primary and Secondary Care (National Clinical Practice Guideline Number 26)*. National Institute for Clinical Excellence (http://guidance.nice.org.uk/CG26/Guidance/pdf/English).

National Institute for Health and Clinical Excellence (2008) *Community Engagement to Improve Health (NICE Public Health Guidance 9)*. NICE (http://www.nice.org.uk/nicemedia/pdf/PH009Guidance.pdf).

Office of the United Nations High Commissioner for Refugees (2011) *UNHCR Global Trends 2010*. UNHCR (http://www.unhcr.org/cgi-bin/texis/vtx/home/opendocPDFViewer.html?docid=4dfa11499).

Rousseau, C. & Measham, T. (2007) Posttraumatic suffering as a source of transformation: a clinical perspective. In *Understanding Trauma: Integrating Biological, Clinical and Cultural Perspectives* (eds L. J. Kirmayer, R. Lemelson & M. Barad), pp. 275–293. Cambridge University Press.

Somasundaram, D. (2007) Collective trauma in northern Sri Lanka: a qualitative psychosocial-ecological study. *International Journal of Mental Health Systems*, **1**:5.

Summerfield, D. (1999) A critique of seven assumptions behind psychological trauma programmes in war affected areas. *Social Science and Medicine*, **48**, 1449–1462.

Tribe, R. & de Silva, P. (1999) Psychological intervention with displaced widows in Sri Lanka. *International Review of Psychiatry*, **11**, 186–192.

United Nations General Assembly (1991) *Strengthening of the Coordination of Humanitarian Emergency Assistance of the United Nations (A/RES/46/182)*. United Nations (http://www.un.org/documents/ga/res/46/a46r182.htm).

Weerackody, C. & Fernando, S. (2011) *Reflections on Mental Health and Well-Being: Learning from Communities Affected by Conflict, Dislocation and Natural Disaster in Sri Lanka*. PRDA.

Wessells, M. (1999) Culture, power and community: intercultural approaches to psychosocial assistance and healing. In *Honoring Differences: Cultural Issues in the Treatment of Trauma and Loss* (eds K. Nader, N. Dubrow & B. Stamm), pp. 267–282. Bruner/Mazel.

Working Group on Children Affected by Armed Conflict and Displacement (1996) *Promoting Psychosocial Well-being among Children Affected by Armed Conflict and Displacement: Principles and Approaches*. International Save the Children Alliance (http://www.savethechildren.org.uk/sites/default/files/docs/psychosocial_care_an_protection_1.pdf).

Yule, W. (ed.) (1999) *Post-Traumatic Stress Disorders: Concepts and Therapy*. John Wiley & Sons.

CHAPTER 2

Will ethnopsychopharmacology lead to changes in clinical practice?

Faisil Sethi

There is much evidence of a variation in the response to psychotropic medications across different ethnic groups, and there are many explanations for this phenomenon. In general, these explanations span three intersecting domains.

The first domain is that related to genetics. Certain patterns of genetic polymorphisms are more or less prevalent in particular ethnic groups. These polymorphisms are known to cause variations in the biological processes underlying the pharmacological actions of psychotropic drugs. The processes of drug metabolism are the primary research area. The second domain relates to the interaction between human biology and the wider environment. For example, enzymes that operate within metabolic pathways can be modulated by factors such as diet, alcohol usage, nicotine, illicit drug use and the use of alternative/complementary therapies. The third domain relates to variations in the expression of mental illness across cultures and ethnicities. This can lead to misdiagnosis, mistreatment and a variation in perceived treatment response. These three domains do not provide a complete explanatory model, but they go some way towards an understanding of the biopsychosociocultural context of psychopharmacotherapy.

This chapter will concentrate on the first domain, that of genetics. I shall start by introducing three areas of scientific endeavour: pharmacogenetics, pharmacokinetics and pharmacodynamics. These three disciplines, taken together in the context of culture and ethnicity, describe the developing field of ethnopsychopharmacology. Pharmacogenetics is the investigation of the genetic factors that influence an individual's reaction to a drug (Arranz *et al*, 2007). Pharmacokinetics is the determination of what happens to the drug in the body; this includes its absorption, distribution, metabolism and excretion. Pharmacodynamics is the study of the biochemical and physiological processes that form the basis for the pharmacological action of a drug, which includes the desired therapeutic effects and the undesired side-effects. The processes involved are complex and often incompletely understood.

Most pharmacogenetic and pharmacokinetic research has focused on the genes encoding the drug-metabolising enzymes. Nearly all psychotropic drugs are metabolised by the cytochrome P450 (CYP) enzymes in the liver (notable exceptions include lithium and lorazepam). The enzymes primarily responsible for psychotropic drug metabolism include CYP1A2, CYP2C19, CYP2D6 and CYP3A4. Genetic polymorphisms exist within all these enzymes, leading to variations of enzyme activity in different populations. Individuals can be characterised as poor, intermediate, extensive or ultra-rapid metabolisers in relation to a particular enzyme, and different populations have different ratios of poor *v.* intermediate *v.* extensive metabolisers (ultra-rapid metabolism is not common) (Lin & Smith, 2000; Arranz *et al*, 2007).

Take the CYP2D6 enzyme as an example: about 7–10% of Caucasians (as categorised in the original publications) are poor metabolisers, 40% are intermediate and 50% are extensive (Kirchheiner *et al*, 2004). Conversely, the prevalence of the poor metaboliser phenotype in Asian populations is around 1%. The dose (of a drug metabolised by CYP2D6) suitable for a White population will often be the normal recommended dose in most Western medical settings; this dose is informed by research which is based primarily on White participants. Yet for an extensive metaboliser, the dose may be too low (leading to reduced efficacy) and for a poor metaboliser the converse may be true, leading to increased side-effects or toxicity. Such effects are much more problematic in drugs with a narrow therapeutic window (e.g. tricyclic antidepressants), and may explain the relative inefficacy or toxicity of certain psychotropic drugs in Black and minority ethnic populations.

The literature is vast and varied, but here are some of the best examples that illustrate a few points. Yue *et al* (1998) demonstrated that the CYP2D6*10 allele in healthy Chinese volunteers led to higher plasma concentrations of the antidepressant nortriptyline because of impaired metabolism. The mutation underlying this genetic variant is over ten times more common in Chinese than in White people. The results of this study indicated that the dose of nortriptyline may need to be lower for Asian than for White patients.

Since the 1980s, there have also been studies that have suggested the need for lower doses of first-generation antipsychotics for Asian than for White people. Most of the studies involved haloperidol, and although the results were far from unequivocal, the take-home message was that serum haloperidol concentrations were higher in Asian than in White patients, hence they may require lower doses (Yu *et al*, 2007; Lambert & Norman, 2008).

More recently, results from the Clinical Antipsychotic Trials of Intervention Effectiveness (CATIE) project (which is sponsored by the US National Institute of Mental Health) showed that the antipsychotic olanzapine cleared 26% faster in patients who identified themselves as Black or African American than in those from other racial and ethnic groups. The estimate for the clearance of the antipsychotic perphenazine was 48% higher in African Americans than in the other racial and ethnic groups. These are not small percentages, and such variable pharmacokinetics can lead to side-effects, toxicity and, consequently, treatment discontinuation. Genetic variations of CYP2D6 have previously been found to be a predictor of perphenazine clearance, and there are known differences in the rates of genetic polymorphism of CYP2D6 between African Americans and other racial and ethnic groups (Bigos *et al*, 2010).

Studies related to pharmacodynamics have concentrated on the components of neurotransmitter systems such as receptors and transporter proteins. The focus for the genetics of antidepressants has been the serotonin and noradrenaline systems, whereas the serotonin and dopamine systems are more relevant for antipsychotics.

A number of studies purport to have found a differential response to a psychotropic due to a genetic variant of a receptor or a transporter protein, with the genetic variant having different frequencies in various ethnic groups. Having said that, the evidence is far from clear. For example, the serotonin transporter gene has a polymorphism within the promoter region which has a long and a short allele. In White people, the short allele is reportedly associated with a poor response to antidepressants of the selective serotonin reuptake inhibitor (SSRI) group, whereas the long allele has a better outcome. However, in a meta-analysis, although Serretti *et al* (2007) confirmed the association of the long allele with better SSRI response, they found the effect to be independent of ethnic differences. To confuse things further, another research group found the opposite to be true in Asians: the short allele was associated with better acute antidepressant response. Thus, the research can paint conflicting pictures.

The key issue is whether ethnopsychopharmacology will lead to changes in clinical practice. Much of the research to date has been marred by low predictive values, which limits its ultimate clinical utility. However, the fast pace at which genetic research has evolved over the past few decades has led to new automated tools to decode the human genome, which has paved the way for much larger studies better able to locate genetic variation. As relevant genes are being identified more accurately, one would expect higher predictive values (Arranz *et al*, 2007).

At the clinical level, one would expect the ethnopsychopharmacological applications to include recommendations on an appropriate therapeutic dose for a psychotropic drug in a particular ethnic group or, more specifically, for a particular type of metaboliser pattern. Combining the evidence available for the major enzymes, a few tests are already available for identifying a person's metaboliser pattern, but these are not in widespread clinical use. There are a number of cytochrome P450 assay services in the UK.

Prediction of treatment response is complex, multigenic and multi-factorial, but a number of genes have been identified that may predict the response to the antipsychotic clozapine with a reasonable degree of accuracy. Genetic tests are available in the UK that report the predictive likelihood that a patient with treatment-resistant schizophrenia will respond to clozapine. Other studies have pointed towards the feasibility of similar genetic tests for the antipsychotics olanzapine and risperidone in the future. Clinically valid pharmacogenetic tools to predict psychiatric treatment response are very much in their infancy.

Predictions of the propensity for a psychotropic drug to produce a particular side-effect are also in the pipeline. A number of genetic polymorphisms have been found that are associated with side-effects such as tardive dyskinesia, weight gain and neuroleptic malignant syndrome (Kirchheiner *et al*, 2004). There are genetic tests currently being developed outside the UK that predict the risk of psychotropic-induced metabolic syndrome.

Ethnopsychopharmacology has its ideals rooted in the move away from a one-size-fits-all approach to a more personalised approach to medicine, which is an underlying driver for pharmacogenetics. However, ethnopsychopharmacology is more than just pharmacogenetics, because it seeks to examine both biological and non-biological variability in pharmacotherapy across ethnicity and culture. The cultural factors include diet, illness behaviour, placebo effects, clinician ideology, and attitudes to medication that shape patients' expectation and adherence. The power of culture to shape treatment response has received little systematic research attention, but it is thought to be extremely important (Lin *et al*, 1999; Smith, 2006).

I advocate that ethnicity and cultural factors should be incorporated into the design and analysis of future trials for new psychotropics and that the evidence from drug trials should be critically appraised through the ethnocultural lens.

The question of clinical utility – for example, whether treatment response or side-effect profiles are different, or whether particular patterns of metabolic activity are more prevalent in particular ethnic groups – requires more coordinated research. Hopefully, such research will provide the evidence base in the future to deal with the wider systemic problem that current clinical guidelines on medications do not always offer the best practice for culturally or ethnically diverse groups.

In essence, there are more questions than answers in the field of ethnopsychopharmacology. We need an international collaborative ethno-psychopharmacology research programme (Ng, 2008).

References

Arranz, M. J., Kerwin, R. W. & Munro, J. C. (2007) Pharmacogenetics and pharmacogenomics in psychiatry: clinical applications. In *Neurogenetics of Psychiatric Disorders* (eds A. Sawa & M. G. McIniss), pp. 173–193. Informa Healthcare USA.

Bigos, K. L., Bies, R. R., Marder, S. R., *et al* (2010) Population pharmacokinetics of antipsychotics. In *Antipsychotic Trials in Schizophrenia: The CATIE Project* (eds T. S. Stroup & J. A. Lieberman), pp. 267–280. Cambridge University Press.

Kirchheiner, J., Nickchen, K., Bauer, M., *et al* (2004) Pharmacogenetics of antidepressants and antipsychotics: the contribution of allelic variations to the phenotype of drug response. *Molecular Psychiatry*, **9**, 442–473.

Lambert, T. & Norman, T. R. (2008) Ethnic differences in psychotropic drug response and pharmacokinetics. In *Ethno-Psychopharmacology: Advances in Current Practice* (eds C. H. Ng, K. Lin & E. Chiu), pp. 38–61. Cambridge University Press.

Lin, K.-M. & Smith, M. W. (2000) Psychopharmacotherapy in the context of culture and ethnicity. In *Ethnicity and Psychopharmacology* (ed. P. Ruiz), pp. 1–36. American Psychiatric Press.

Lin, K.-M., Smith, M. W. & Mendoza, R. P. (1999) Psychopharmacology in cross cultural psychiatry. In *Cross Cultural Psychiatry* (eds J. M. Herrera, W. B. Lawson & J. J. Sramek), pp. 45–52. John Wiley & Sons.

Ng, C. H. (2008) Research directions in ethno-psychopharmacology. In *Ethno-Psychopharmacology: Advances in Current Practice* (eds C. H. Ng, K. Lin & E. Chiu), pp. 169–176. Cambridge University Press.

Serretti, M. K., Kato, M., Ronchi, D. D., *et al* (2007) Meta-analysis of serotonin transporter gene promoter polymorphism (5-HTTLPR) association with selective serotonin reuptake inhibitor efficacy in depressed patients. *Molecular Psychiatry*, **12**, 247–257.

Smith, M. W. (2006) Ethnopsychopharmacology. In *Clinical Manual of Cultural Psychiatry* (ed. R. F. Lim), pp. 207–235. American Psychiatric Publishing.

Yu, S., Liu, S. & Lin, K. (2007) Psychopharmacology across cultures. In *Textbook of Cultural Psychiatry* (eds D. Bhugra & K. Bhui), pp. 402–413. Cambridge University Press.

Yue, Q., Zhong, Z., Tybring, G., *et al* (1998) Pharmacokinetics of nortriptyline and its 10-hydroxy metabolite in Chinese subjects of different CYP2D6 genotypes. *Clinical Pharmacology & Therapeutics*, **64**, 384–390.

CHAPTER 3

Does cognitive–behavioural therapy work for people with very different cultural orientations and backgrounds?

Shanaya Rathod, Farooq Naeem and David Kingdon

Cognitive–behavioural therapy (CBT) can be used across cultures, but only if appropriately adapted (Rathod *et al*, 2010). A personalised and pragmatic therapy, CBT uses reasoning to provide a conceptual framework of mental illness that is not inconsistent with Eastern and other philosophies (Rathod & Kingdon, 2009). The client (patient) and therapist develop a collaborative understanding of the client's perceived problems, so that a mutually respectful exploration of the problem can be developed to work on the issues identified (Bhui & Bhugra, 2004). The collaborative approach allows the patient to take an active role as an expert of their own culture and the therapist to personalise the therapy to the patient's needs.

People with depressive illness and anxiety usually have beliefs about the self, others and the world that are unhelpful. Cognitive–behavioural therapy involves exploration of these core beliefs and attempts to modify them, and there is a strong focus on involvement of the patient in the therapeutic process. However, core beliefs, underlying assumptions and even the content of automatic thoughts might vary with culture (Padesky & Greenberger, 1995). The practice of CBT without adaptation in minority groups can adversely affect the therapeutic alliance between patient and therapist and risks disengagement of patients from therapy (Rathod *et al*, 2005). In patients, this can lead to disappointment and loss of hope, particularly as people from ethnic minority groups are less likely to trust mental health services in the first place (Thornicroft *et al*, 1999). In therapists, a patient's disengagement might leave them feeling incompetent, especially if they do not understand the cultural issues involved.

Griner & Smith (2006), in their meta-analysis, provided suggestive evidence that culturally adapted interventions are effective. Some findings pointed to the possibility that clients who had the greatest need for accommodations (i.e. poorly acculturated, non-English-speaking adults) received the greatest benefit from such adaptations. Small pilots from many cultural groups have found adapted CBT to be successful in ethnic minority populations (Patel *et al*, 2007; Rojas *et al*, 2007; Rahman *et al*, 2008). Muñoz and colleagues have conducted a number of studies on the cultural adaptation of CBT for the treatment and prevention of depression in adults from ethnic minority groups in the USA (e.g. Kohn *et al*, 2002; Miranda *et al*, 2003; Muñoz & Mendelson, 2005). For example, Kohn *et al* (2002) compared standard group CBT with adapted group CBT for African American women presenting with major depression and reported positive results for the adapted therapy. In Pakistan, Naeem *et al* (2009) have adapted CBT for depression, with promising results.

Various cognitive therapists from the USA have described their experience of working with Native Americans, Alaska Natives, Latinos and Latinas, African Americans, Asian Americans, people of Arab heritage and Orthodox Jews (Hays & Imasama, 2006). Pamela Hays has offered a framework for therapists using CBT with ethnic minority clients that can be remembered by the acronym ADDRESSING and consists of the following areas of importance: (A) age and generational influences, (D) developmental or acquired (D) disabilities, (R) religion and spiritual orientation, (E) ethnicity, (S) socioeconomic status, (S) sexual orientation, (I) indigenous heritage, (N) national origin and (G) gender (Hays & Imasama, 2006).

There are challenges in adapting CBT to different cultures. In therapy, information on current thought and beliefs and how they were arrived at is assembled into a 'formulation'. This draws together predisposing, precipitating, perpetuating and protective factors with current and underlying concerns about interactions between thoughts, feelings and behaviours. Cultural orientation influences psychopathology, illness attributions, help-seeking behaviours, care pathways and barriers to engaging with therapy. Being aware of patients' beliefs about their illness, its causes and its treatment are important. For example, some attribute mental illness to magical beings such as jinn, evil spirits or demons, others to a curse or spell cast by a person. In South Asian Muslim communities, such casting of an evil eye is called *Nazar lagana*, in some African–Caribbean communities it is *Obeah* (Rathod *et al*, 2010). Some patients present with somatic complaints when mentally unwell, and the therapist needs to focus on these physical symptoms in order to engage the individual before exploring their mental distress. Exploring patients' views, their knowledge of therapy and their expectations of it can provide valuable information. Therefore, including spiritual and cultural explanations in the formulation is important. Adaptation requires authentic conceptualisation of a particular culture in the design of the adapted therapy, acknowledgement of the relevance of culture (Frankish *et al*, 2007) and the ability to generalise between subgroups.

Experience suggests that therapy techniques also need adjustments. Language is the main tool used to deliver a psychotherapy and therefore any adaptation must include culturally sensitive translation of therapeutic concepts. Communication styles might be different and assertiveness techniques may need to be adapted. People from Asian cultures are often not comfortable using assertive communication with elders or with those in authority. When working with South Asian Muslims, a directive style of therapy might be preferable to a collaborative style. The involvement of family in an individual's therapy may be more important for clients from non-Western cultures. Engaging family members can bring certain strengths to therapy, such as improvements in follow-up and greater adherence to homework assignments (Naeem *et al*, 2009; Rathod *et al*, 2010).

Barriers in healthcare systems, for example a lack of resources, insufficient trained therapists and the distance between the patient's home and the health centre, are important considerations when discussing the success of CBT in different countries. In non-Western and low- and middle-income countries, it is common for patients to travel long distances for treatment. Attending weekly or sometimes even monthly sessions might not be possible for some.

In working with immigrant populations, therapy needs to be adjusted to accommodate the extent to which the patient is aligned to their minority culture in the process of acculturation. Therapists need to assess their patient's acculturation to Western culture, as this will have implications for the level of adaptations necessary to achieve a positive outcome (Rathod *et al*, 2010).

A non-judgemental approach, appraisal of culturally tuned cognitive biases, addressing prejudices and shame, awareness of gender and the role of family, use of validation and mindfulness, awareness of religion and its role, and modification of language: all are strategies to keep in mind in practising psychotherapy with clients of a different culture.

In the UK and many other countries, CBT is the most widely recommended psychological therapy for most mental health problems, including depression, anxiety, obsessive–compulsive disorder and psychosis (e.g. National Collaborating Centre for Mental Health, 2009). Yet little attention has been given to modifying and adapting its therapeutic framework and practice (Williams *et al*, 2006) to make it meaningful and compatible with diverse ethnic, cultural and religious contexts (Rathod *et al*, 2008). With the increasing dissemination of cognitive therapy across widely diverse cultures around the world (Casas, 1988; Williams *et al*, 2006; Chen *et al*, 2007), this has become a matter of priority, as the current evidence base boasts very few adequately powered randomised trials of CBT in which specific ethnic groups are included in sufficient numbers to assess treatment efficacy and effectiveness.

References and further reading

Bhui, K. & Bhugra, D. (2004) Communication with patients from other cultures: the place of explanatory models. *Advances in Psychiatric Treatment*, **10**, 474–478.

Casas, J. M. (1988) Cognitive behavioral approaches: a minority perspective. *Counseling Psychologist*, **16**, 106–110.

Castro, F. G., Barrera Jr., M. & Steiker, L. K. H. (2010) Issues and challenges in the design of culturally adapted evidence-based interventions. *Annual Review of Clinical Psychology*, **6**, 213–239.

Chen, J., Nakano, Y., Ietzugu, T., *et al* (2007) Group cognitive behaviour therapy for Japanese patients with social anxiety disorder: preliminary outcomes and their predictors. *BMC Psychiatry*, **7**, 69.

Frankish, C. J., Lovatto, C. Y. & Poureslami, I. (2007) Models, theories, and principles of health promotion. In *Health Promotion in Multicultural Populations: A Handbook for Practitioners and Students* (eds M. V. Kline & R. M. Huff), pp. 57–101. Sage Publications.

Griner, D. & Smith, T. B. (2006) Culturally adapted mental health interventions: a meta-analytic review. *Psychotherapy: Theory, Research and Practice*, **43**, 531–548.

Hays, P. & Imasama, G. Y. (2006) *Culturally Responsive Cognitive–Behavioral Therapy: Assessment, Practice and Supervision*. American Psychological Association.

Kohn, L. P., Oden, T., Muñoz, R. F., *et al* (2002) Adapted cognitive behavioral group therapy for depressed low-income African American women. *Community Mental Health Journal*, **38**, 497–504.

Miranda, J., Azocar, F., Organista, K., *et al* (2003) Treatment of depression among impoverished primary care patients from ethnic minority groups. *Psychiatric Services*, **54**, 219–225.

Muñoz, R. F. & Mendelson, T. (2005) Toward evidence-based interventions for diverse populations: the San Francisco General Hospital prevention and treatment manuals. *Journal of Consulting and Clinical Psychology*, **73**, 790–799.

Naeem, F., Ayub, M., Gobbi, M., *et al* (2009) Development of Southampton Adaptation Framework for CBT (SAF-CBT): a framework for adaptation of CBT in non-western culture. *Journal of the Pakistan Psychiatric Society*, **6**, 79–84.

Naeem, F., Phiri, P., Rathod, S., *et al* (2010) Using CBT with diverse patients: working with South Asian Muslims. In *Oxford Guide to Surviving as a CBT Therapist* (eds M. Mueller, H. Kennerley, F. McManus, *et al*), pp. 41–56. Oxford University Press.

National Collaborating Centre for Mental Health (2009) *Schizophrenia: Core Interventions in the Treatment and Management of Schizophrenia in Adults in Primary and Secondary Care (NICE Clinical Guideline 82)*. National Institute for Health and Clinical Excellence (http://www.nice.org.uk/nicemedia/pdf/CG82NICEGuideline.pdf).

Padesky, C. & Greenberger, D. (1995) *Clinician's Guide to Mind over Mood*. Guilford Press.

Patel, V., Araya, R., Chatterjee, S., *et al* (2007) Treatment and prevention of mental disorders in low-income and middle-income countries. *Lancet*, **370**, 991–1005.

Rahman, A., Malik, A., Sikander, S., *et al* (2008) Cognitive behaviour therapy-based intervention by community health workers for mothers with depression and their infants in rural Pakistan: a cluster-randomised controlled trial. *Lancet*, **372**, 902–909.

Rathod, S. & Kingdon, D. (2009) Cognitive behaviour therapy across cultures. *Psychiatry*, **8**, 370–371.

Rathod, S., Kingdon, D., Smith, P., *et al* (2005) Insight into schizophrenia: the effects of cognitive behavioural therapy on the components of insight and association with sociodemographics: data on a previously published randomised controlled trial. *Schizophrenia Research*, **74**, 211–219.

Rathod, S., Naeem, F., Phiri, P., *et al* (2008) Expansion of psychological therapies. *British Journal of Psychiatry*, **193**, 256–257.

Rathod, S., Phiri, P., Kingdon, D., *et al* (2010) Developing culturally sensitive cognitive behaviour therapy for psychosis for ethnic minority patients by exploration and incorporation of service users' and health professionals' views and opinions. *Behavioural and Cognitive Psychotherapies*, **38**, 511–533.

Rojas, G., Fritsch, R., Solis, J., *et al* (2007) Treatment of postnatal depression in low-income mothers in primary-care clinics in Santiago, Chile: a randomised controlled trial. *Lancet*, **370**, 1629–1637.

Thornicroft, G., Parkman, S. & Ruggeri, M. (1999) Satisfaction with mental health services: issues for ethnic minorities. In *Ethnicity: An Agenda for Mental Health* (eds D. Bhugra & V. Bahl), pp. 158–165. Gaskell.

Williams, M. W., Koong, H. & Haarhoff, B. (2006) Cultural considerations in using cognitive behaviour therapy with Chinese people: a case study of an elderly Chinese woman with generalised anxiety disorder. *New Zealand Journal of Psychology*, **35**, 153–162.

CHAPTER 4

Can you do meaningful cognitive–behavioural therapy through an interpreter?

Shanaya Rathod and Farooq Naeem

There is evidence that when interpreters are necessary and used well and appropriately in therapy, the benefits for both client and therapist include greater understanding, better engagement and more accurate cooperation (Faust & Drickey, 1986; Tribe, 1999). D'Ardenne *et al* (2007) report that cognitive–behavioural therapy (CBT) resulted in significant improvements in routine clinical outcomes of three groups of patients with post-traumatic stress disorder: refugees who required interpreters; refugees who did not require interpreters; and English-speaking non-refugees.

The pragmatic approach of CBT, especially the option to use its behavioural component rather than techniques such as Socratic dialogue and the downward arrow procedure (vertical descent technique), make it possible to conduct CBT successfully through interpreters.

The role of the interpreter in therapy is complex and there have been many debates about the interpreter's effect on the therapeutic alliance, empathy and transference. Orlinsky *et al* (1994) see therapy through interpreters as a group process, whereas Raval (2003) describes the interpreter as potentially encompassing the roles of translator, bilingual co-worker, cultural broker, cultural consultant, advocate for the service user, intermediary, conciliator, community advocate and link worker. At their worst, therapy sessions conducted through an interpreter can be described as the blind leading the blind; at their best, the interpreter can help understanding and enhance the therapeutic relationship. Fear of breach of confidentiality, especially if the interpreter is from the patient's community, has been voiced; and if a family member takes on the interpreting role, there are often many conflicts of interest (Rathod *et al*, 2010).

Factors that determine the type of interaction and success of interpreted CBT

The training and experience of the interpreter is an important consideration. In the successful study mentioned above (d'Ardenne *et al*, 2007), the interpreters had at least 1 year's experience in healthcare interpreting. The researchers closely matched patients to interpreters in terms of gender, ethnicity and any political sensitivity, and the same interpreter was used throughout treatment, unless the patient requested a different one. Untrained and inexperienced interpreters, such as family members, friends or support staff, make more errors in interpreting, and the use of trained professional interpreters and bilingual healthcare providers can improve patient satisfaction, quality of care and outcomes (Flores, 2005). A large multicentre study in the USA assessed how Chinese and Vietnamese patients with limited English proficiency rated the communication and quality of healthcare they received during clinic visits. Patients who communicated with their clinicians through qualified interpreters gave ratings similar to those of patients who saw clinicians who spoke their language. However, where an interpreter was used, patients' evaluation of overall quality of care were strongly associated with the quality of the interpreter (Green *et al*, 2005).

Preparation and goal-setting with the interpreter are key determinants of success in interpreted therapy. Developing a strong and effective working relationship between the clinician and the interpreter is essential. Regular meetings between the interpreter and the clinician before and after therapy sessions are advised, for discussion of therapy material and the goals of the session (Stansfield, 1981). Rules of confidentiality and the remit of the interpreter should be agreed. This ensures that both are working with mutual understanding and codes of conduct.

The therapist should clarify the role of the interpreter at the start of therapy. It is inevitable that the interpreter will influence sessions. It is essential for the therapist to recognise the complexity of the interpreter's task, particularly the power that interpreters have to control the information being relayed back and forth and thus influence the outcome of the intervention. There is a risk that interpreters may dissuade patients from giving, or may fail to convey, information seen as stigmatising to their culture or religion (Putch, 1985; Westermeyer, 1990). Some therapists think of interpreters as machines that merely translate, without interpretation of the cultural context. However, for therapy to be successful, the interpreter's role in it has to be recognised as an integral part of a three-person alliance, with the interpreter viewed also as a witness to clients' stories, experience and trust (Miller *et al*, 2005). The therapist has to accept the concept of an interpreter who actively delivers the message and practises an interactive model of interpreting.

In interpreted therapy, it is important for the therapist to be attentive to the patient, to address them directly and to observe non-verbal clues and body language between questions. Use of simple language and clarification of any confusing non-verbal gestures is useful. Appropriate metaphors, symbols and idioms might help with engagement in therapy. These things require that adequate time is allowed for preparation and delivery of sessions, which may take twice as long.

Negatives of using interpreters in psychiatry have been described, such as interpreters breaking confidentiality or not translating all material (Westermeyer, 1990). Other problems include omission, addition, condensing, substitution, role exchange and normalisation – all of which would be important in CBT. The very presence of an interpreter, their movements and facial expressions, can interfere with the therapeutic process, causing the patient to alter the form and content of what they say, while the process of interpreting can interrupt flow of sessions (Farooq *et al*, 1997). Therapists must understand the potential negative effects that this can have on the process of therapy and address them early.

On balance, meaningful CBT can be delivered through interpreters, because of the pragmatic and flexible nature of the therapy. Interpreters should be selected with care, and supervision is recommended for all interpreters working in therapy sessions. They should receive additional support in difficult or distressing cases. It is advisable to have consistency and continuity of supervision and support (Tribe & Morrissey, 2004). Preparation, awareness of pitfalls and attentiveness to non-verbal clues are other key determinants of success. Tribe & Thompson (2008) have made recommendations for the provision of interpreted psychological therapies and provide a guide for psychologists working with the help of interpreters. However, this is an area that has implications for service providers and service commissioners, and that merits further research.

References and further reading

D'Ardenne, P., Ruaro, L., Cestari, L., *et al* (2007) Does interpreter-mediated CBT with traumatized refugee people work? A comparison of patient outcomes in east London. *Behavioural and Cognitive Psychotherapy*, **35**, 293–301.

Farooq, S., Fear, C. F. & Oyebode, F. (1997) An investigation of the adequacy of psychiatric interviews conducted through an interpreter. *Psychiatric Bulletin*, **21**, 209–213.

Faust, S. & Drickey, R. (1986) Working with interpreters. *Journal of Family Practice*, **22**, 131–138.

Flores, G. (2005) The impact of medical interpreter services on the quality of health care: a systematic review. *Medical Care Research and Review*, **62**, 255–299.

Green, A. R., Ngo-Metzger, Q., Legedza, A. T. R., *et al* (2005) Interpreter services, language concordance, and health care quality: experiences of Asian Americans with limited English proficiency. *Journal of General Internal Medicine*, **20**, 1050–1056.

Hamerdinger, S. & Ben, K. (2003) Therapy using interpreters: questions on the use of interpreters in therapeutic settings for monolingual therapists. *Journal of the American Deafness and Rehabilitation Association*, **36** (3), 12–30.

Miller, K., Martell, Z. L., Pazdirek, L., *et al* (2005) The role of interpreters in psychotherapy with refugees: an exploratory study. *American Journal of Orthopsychiatry*, **75**, 27–39.

Munday, A. (2009) *The Impact of Interpreters in Therapy with Refugees* (Doctoral Thesis). University of Birmingham Research Archive.

Ngo-Metzger, Q., Sorkin, D. H., Phillips, R. S., *et al* (2007) Providing high-quality care for limited English proficient patients: the importance of language concordance and interpreter use. *Journal of General Internal Medicine*, **22** (suppl. 2), 324–330.

Orlinsky, D., Grawe, K. & Parks, B. (1994) Process and outcome in psychotherapy – *noch einmal*. In *Handbook of Psychotherapy and Behavior Change* (4th edn) (eds A. E. Bergin & S. L. Garfield), pp. 270–378. John Wiley & Sons.

Putch, R. W. (1985) Cross-cultural communication: the special case of interpreters in health care. *JAMA*, **254**, 3344–3348.

Rathod, S., Phiri, P., Kingdon, D., *et al* (2010) Developing culturally sensitive cognitive behaviour therapy for psychosis for ethnic minority patients by exploration and incorporation of service users' and health professionals' views and opinions. *Journal of Behavioural and Cognitive Psychotherapies*, **38**, 511–533.

Raval, H. (2003) An overview of the issues in the work with interpreters. In *Working with Interpreters in Mental Health* (eds R. Tribe & H. Raval), pp. 8–29. Brunner-Routledge.

Stansfield, M. (1981) Psychological issues in mental health interpreting. *Journal of Interpretation*, **1**, 18–31.

Tribe, R. (1999) Bridging the gap or damming the flow? Some observations on using interpreters/bicultural workers when working with refugee clients, many of whom have been tortured. *British Journal of Medical Psychology*, **72**, 567–576.

Tribe, R. & Morrissey, J. (2004) Good practice issues in working with interpreters in mental health. *Intervention*, **2**, 129–142.

Tribe, R. & Thompson, K. (2008) *Working with Interpreters in Health Settings: Guidelines for Psychologists*. British Psychological Society.

Westermeyer, J. (1990) Working with an interpreter in psychiatric assessment and treatment. *Journal of Nervous and Mental Disease*, **178**, 745–749.

Zayas, L. H., Cabassa, L. J., Perez, M. C., *et al* (2007) Using interpreters in diagnostic research and practice: pilot results and recommendations. *Journal of Clinical Psychiatry*, **68**, 924–928.

CHAPTER 5

Are particular psychotherapeutic orientations indicated with specific ethnic minority groups?

Adil Qureshi

Matching the type of psychological intervention to specific conditions or symptom profiles is gaining increasing popularity, particularly in light of the emphasis on evidence-based medicine and managed care (Barlow, 2004). It may also be the case that cultural differences in the expression and expected management of distress are such that certain cultural groups may derive greater benefit from specific types of psychotherapeutic approach or orientation. This chapter explores these clinical options.

Cultural values and specific therapeutic approaches

Directive approaches

Prince (2004) has described his very unsuccessful experience of applying insight and non-directive therapeutic techniques with the Yoruba in Nigeria in the early 1960s. He concluded that, given the cultural values of the Yoruba, a focus on psychological self-awareness and on childhood experiences, utilising open-ended questions in which the patient is invited to take the lead, is simply inapplicable and, indeed, counterproductive. A number of multiculturalists follow the same notion, arguing that various non-Western groups prefer or derive greater benefit from directive types of therapy, because of characteristics – perhaps world views – specific to the culture in question (Lin & Cheung, 1999; Sue & Sue, 1999).

Many non-Western cultures prefer an action orientation, look to the clinician as the expert and consider the expression (and recognition) of emotion, if at all, to belong to the domain of close family members. Such may be the strength of these characteristics that, as Prince suggested, individuals will be inimical to exploration of insight and emotional processes, and will vastly prefer and benefit from directive approaches (Atkinson & Lowe, 1996; Sue & Sue, 1999; Kirmayer, 2007). Research shows that cognitive–behavioural therapy, with or without cultural adaptation, is effective with ethnic minority and immigrant patients (Miranda *et al*, 2003, 2005; Voss Horrell, 2008).

Relational approaches

Relational psychoanalysts have argued that their approach, with its thematisation of a 'three-person model' in which the clinician, patient and overall social context are all included, is particularly valuable for individuals from collectivist cultures, given the focus in these cultures on interpersonal relationships (Perez-Foster *et al*, 1996; Altman, 1999; Walls, 2004; Moran, 2006). Not only are such treatment orientations adaptable to other sorts of selves (there is a strong concordance between the relational and sociocentric self); also, the overt inclusion of the social context situates mental distress within the sociopolitical dynamics that affect patients. These include institutional racism, as well as power and privilege differentials between clinician and patient. Kakar (2006), a psychoanalyst from India, makes the argument that, with its focus on transference and countertransference, a relational phenomenon, psychoanalysis is very adaptable to effective work with patients from different cultures. Interpersonal psychotherapy is effective with Latin American immigrants, it is argued, because of the value Latin cultures place on social relations, through which distress is experienced, expressed and can be ameliorated (Rosselló & Bernal, 1999; Miranda *et al*, 2005; Rosselló *et al*, 2008).

Thompson (1989) criticises the notion that people from ethnic minorities are not amenable to psychoanalysis (are unanalysable) as being racist, predicated on the prejudice that they are limited in their capacity for insight, self-awareness and a depth orientation. At the same time, some analysts argue that self-disclosure, self-awareness and a psychological orientation are particularly Western middle-class values and, as such, not appropriate foci of treatment in other groups (Sue & Sue, 1999). Kakar (2006) challenges this notion and identifies self-awareness as a fundamental Hindu value. In addition, the Koran states, 'He who knows himself knows God', which suggests, perhaps, that the issue at hand may not be the psychological orientation or insight of the patient, but rather the psychotherapeutic process itself or the approach used by the clinician.

Level of therapeutic intervention

The matching of therapeutic approach according to culture is largely predicated on notions of static and stable cultural values or meaning systems. Kirmayer, however, presents the very interesting idea that there are different sorts of 'self' (Kirmayer, 2007). Therefore, the optimal treatment approach will depend on the patient's primary, most prominent or most visible epistemic perspective and/or value orientations. To that end, people from individualistic cultures will be best served by conventional approaches, which are individualistic, whereas people from collectivistic cultures benefit most from a therapeutic orientation that works at the family level, such as family therapy (McGoldrick *et al*, 2005). Examples from French ethnopsychiatry tested individual therapy but in a group setting that included family members, medical interpreters and/or intercultural mediators, and additional therapists (perhaps from the culture of origin of the patient). The idea is that, in certain cultures, an individual's problems are best solved in a communal context (Sturm *et al*, 2008, 2010).

Indigenous and culture-specific therapies

It can be argued that conventional psychotherapies are Western or modernist creations, and as such are Eurocentric and thus of limited, if any, applicability to those from other cultural backgrounds (Moghaddam, 1993; Parker, 1998). Proponents of such a perspective argue for a more culture-specific approach and that indigenous psychologies, adaptations of traditional healing, or therapies designed for the culture in question are more appropriate (Moghaddam, 1993; Moodley & West, 2005; Allwood & Berry, 2006). Examples of this include Morita therapy from Japan (Fujita, 1986), Cuento therapy from Latin America (Costantino *et al*, 1986) and Afrocentric therapy for African Americans (Phillips, 1990). Moodley & West (2005) give a comprehensive overview of different indigenous approaches.

It is not the therapeutic approach but rather the meta-theory that needs adaptation

Cultural competence

Many multiculturalists, although critical of conventional Eurocentric approaches, consider that some sort of modification can make them effective for other cultures. One response operates at a meta-theoretical level, involving significant shifts in the therapist's skills, knowledge and attitudes so as to achieve cultural sensitivity and competence in the therapeutic endeavour (Sue *et al*, 1996; Arredondo & Arciniega, 2001; Coleman, 2004; Goh, 2005; Moodley & Palmer, 2006; Bezanson & James, 2007). Although the cultural competence movement has gained considerable attention and success, counselling and therapy tend to be process oriented and there is little in the way of empirical evidence demonstrating the effectiveness of the approach (Vega, 2005; Bhui *et al*, 2007; Qureshi *et al*, 2008).

Cultural adaptations

With the growing focus on evidence-based medicine, a number of multiculturalists have opted for marrying empirically supported treatment approaches with cultural sensitivity, which has resulted in the cultural adaptation movement (Lau, 2006; Bernal *et al*, 2009). This provides a specific means by which to adapt empirically supported treatments to the cultural values and context of different ethnic groups. Receiving increased attention, this approach has also come under some criticism. LaRoche & Christopher (2008) state that standard incorporation of race and ethnicity into empirically supported treatment research is deficient in that it artificially collapses into a single construct considerable racial and ethnic diversity. To that end, it is a matter not of establishing which therapeutic approaches are most suitable for which ethnic groups, but rather of using a framework in which to take into consideration interactions between the patient's (cultural) aptitude and the treatment approach (Beutler *et al*, 2000). This takes an ideographic approach, looking at the patient with greater specificity within his or her specific cultural context. Wong *et al* (2007) tested this very idea and found that preference among Asian patients for directive therapy was moderated by each individual's expectations of treatment. From this perspective, *a priori* determination of which therapeutic approach is most appropriate without taking the specific individual into consideration, regardless of cultural origin, is incoherent.

Psychological v. structural approaches

Psychotherapy runs the real risk of imposing or indeed promoting the sort of self in the patient that is functional in the dominant socioeconomic system. Psychotherapeutic approaches may be characterised by an implicit (or not so implicit) ideology. Unadapted therapeutic approaches certainly run this risk, but it is uncertain the degree to which adapted or indigenous therapies also inadvertently impose a particular self that is not closely matched to that of the patient. For example, a strategic family therapy promoted by Kim (1985) for use with Asian families does not challenge existing power structures within the family. Yet, this may be necessary at times if that power structure is a source of the patient's distress.

The notion that therapeutic approaches need to be adapted, developed or supplemented is predicated on the idea that conventional therapeutic approaches are indeed Eurocentric and that this is unhelpful; that these approaches have embedded within them the values of the dominant group, of the *status quo*, which does not permit structural factors in society to be identified as pathogenic (Sue *et al*, 1996; Rose, 1998; Walcott, 2006). So psychotherapy may serve only to reproduce existing power relations by situating suffering within the individual, rather than in their sociopolitical context – a context that will be normative for some but not for others (Rose, 1998; Walls, 2004). Consequently, some call for a therapy of liberation that specifically focuses on structural issues related to the patient's sociopolitical context (Atkinson *et al*, 1993; Essandoh, 1996; Burton & Kagan, 2005).

References

Allwood, C. M. & Berry, J. W. (2006) Origins and development of indigenous psychologies: an international analysis. *International Journal of Psychology*, **41**, 243–268.

Altman, N. (1999) Psychoanalytic perspective on clinical work in the inner city. In *Psychoanalytic Therapy as Health Care: Effectiveness and Economics in the 21st Century* (eds H. Kaley, M. N. Eagle & D. L. Wolitzky), pp. 257–271. Analytic Press.

Arredondo, P. & Arciniega, M. G. (2001) Strategies and techniques for counselor training based on the Multicultural Counseling Competencies. *Journal of Mental Health Counseling*, **29**, 263–274.

Atkinson, D. R. & Lowe, S. M. (1996) The role of ethnicity, cultural knowledge, and conventional techniques in counseling and psychotherapy. In *Handbook of Multicultural Counseling* (eds J. G. Ponterotto, J. M. Casas, L. A. Suzuki, *et al*), pp. 387–414. Sage.

Atkinson, D. R., Thompson, C. E. & Grant, S. K. (1993) A three-dimensional model for counseling racial/ethnic minorities. *Counseling Psychologist*, **21**, 257–277.

Barlow, D. H. (2004) Psychological treatments. *American Psychologist*, **59**, 869–878.

Bernal, G., Jiménez-Chafey, M. I. & Domenech Rodríguez, M. M. (2009) Cultural adaptation of treatments: a resource for considering culture in evidence-based practice. *Professional Psychology: Research and Practice*, **40**, 361–368.

Beutler, L. E., Clarkin, J. F. & Bongar, B. M. (2000) *Guidelines for the Systematic Treatment of the Depressed Patient*. Oxford University Press.

Bezanson, B. & James, S. (2007) Culture-general and culture-specific approaches to counselling: complementary stances. *International Journal for the Advancement of Counselling*, **29**, 159–171.

Bhui, K., Warfa, N., Edonya, P., *et al* (2007) Cultural competence in mental health care: a review of model evaluations. *BMC Health Services Research*, **7**, 15.

Burton, M. & Kagan, C. (2005) Liberation social psychology: learning from Latin America. *Journal of Community & Applied Social Psychology*, **15**, 63–78.

Coleman, H. L. K. (2004) Multicultural counseling competencies in a pluralistic society. *Journal of Mental Health Counseling*, **26**, 56–66.

Costantino, G., Malgady, R. G. & Rogler, L. H. (1986) Cuento therapy: a culturally sensitive modality for Puerto Rican children. *Journal of Consulting and Clinical Psychology*, **54**, 639–645.

Essandoh, P. K. (1996) Multicultural counseling as the "fourth force". *Counseling Psychologist*, **24**, 126–137.

Fujita, C. (1986) *Morita Therapy*. Igaku-Shoin.

Goh, M. (2005) Cultural competence and master therapists: an inextricable relationship. *Journal of Mental Health Counseling*, **27**, 71–82.

Kakar, S. (2006) Culture and psychoanalysis: a personal journey. *Social Analysis*, **50**, 25–44.

Kim, S. (1985) Family therapy for Asian Americans: a strategic-structural framework. *Psychotherapy*, **22**, 342–348.

Kirmayer, L. J. (2007) Psychotherapy and the cultural concept of the person. *Transcultural Psychiatry*, **44**, 232–257.

La Roche, M. & Christopher, M. S. (2008) Culture and empirically supported treatments: on the road to a collision? *Culture & Psychology*, **14**, 333–356.

Lau, A. S. (2006) Making the case for selective and directed cultural adaptations of evidence-based treatments: examples from parent training. *Clinical Psychology: Science and Practice*, **13**, 295–310.

Lin, K.-M. & Cheung, F. (1999) Mental health issues for Asian Americans. *Psychiatric Services*, **50**, 774–780.

McGoldrick, M., Giordano, J. & Garcia-Preto, N. (2005) *Ethnicity and Family Therapy*. Guilford Press.

Miranda, J., Chung, J. Y., Green, B. L., *et al* (2003) Treating depression in predominantly low-income young minority women. *JAMA*, **290**, 57–65.

Miranda, J., Bernal, G., Lau, A., *et al* (2005) State of the science on psychosocial interventions for ethnic minorities. *Annual Review of Clinical Psychology*, **1**, 113–142.

Moghaddam, F. M. (1993) Traditional and modern psychologies in competing cultural systems: lessons from Iran 1978–81. In *Indigenous Psychologies: Research and Experience in Cultural Context* (eds U. Kim & J. W. Berry), pp. 118–132. Sage.

Moodley, R. & Palmer, S. (2006) *Race, Culture and Psychotherapy: Critical Perspectives in Multicultural Practice*. Routledge.

Moodley, R. & West, W. (2005) *Integrating Traditional Healing Practices into Counseling and Psychotherapy*. Sage.

Moran, J. C. (2006) *Dialogues on Difference: Studies of Diversity in the Therapeutic Relationship*. APA Press.

Parker, I. (1998) Against postmodernism. *Theory & Psychology*, **8**, 601–627.

Perez-Foster, R. A., Moskowitz, M. & Javier, R. A. (1996) *Reaching across Boundaries of Culture and Class*. Jason Aronson.

Phillips, F. (1990) NTU psychotherapy: an Afrocentric approach. *Journal of Black Psychology*, **17**, 215–222.

Prince, R. (2004) Western psychotherapy and the Yoruba: problems of insight and nondirective technique. In *Handbook of Culture, Therapy and Healing* (eds U. P. Gielen, J. M. Fish & J. G. Draguns), pp. 311–320. Lawrence Erlbaum Associates.

Qureshi, A., Collazos, F., Ramos, M., *et al* (2008) Cultural competency training in psychiatry. *European Psychiatry*, **23**, 49–58.

Rose, N. (1998) *Inventing our Selves: Psychology, Power, and Personhood*. Cambridge University Press.

Rosselló, J. & Bernal, G. (1999) The efficacy of cognitive–behavioral and interpersonal treatments for depression in Puerto Rican adolescents. *Journal of Consulting and Clinical Psychology*, **67**, 734–745.

Rosselló, J., Bernal, G. & Rivera-Medina, C. (2008) Individual and group CBT and IPT for Puerto Rican adolescents with depressive symptoms. *Cultural Diversity and Ethnic Minority Psychology*, **14**, 234–245.

Sturm, G., Heidenreich, F. & Moro, M. R. (2008) Transcultural clinical work with immigrants, asylum seekers and refugees at Avicenne Hospital, France. *International Journal of Migration, Health and Social Care*, **4**, 33–40.

Sturm, G., Nadig, M. & Moro, M. R. (2010) Writing therapies – an ethnographic approach to transcultural therapies. *Forum: Qualitative Social Research/Sozialforschung*, **11** (3) Art. 1.

Sue, D. W. & Sue, D. (1999) *Counseling the Culturally Different: Theory and Practice* (3rd edn). John Wiley & Sons.

Sue, D. W., Ivey, A. E. & Pederson, P. B. (1996) *Theory of Multicultural Counseling and Therapy*. Brooks/Cole.

Thompson, C. L. (1989) Psychoanalytic psychotherapy with inner city patients. *Journal of Contemporary Psychotherapy*, **19**, 137–148.

Vega, W. A. (2005) Higher stakes ahead for cultural competence. *General Hospital Psychiatry*, **27**, 446–450.

Voss Horrell, S. C. (2008) Effectiveness of cognitive–behavioral therapy with adult ethnic minority clients: a review. *Professional Psychology: Research and Practice*, **39**, 160–168.

Walcott, R. (2006) Multiculturally crazy: diagnosis in Black. In *Race, Culture and Psychotherapy: Critical Perspectives in Multicultural Practice* (eds R. Moodley & S. Palmer), pp. 27–35. Routledge.

Walls, G. B. (2004) Toward a critical global psychoanalysis. *Psychoanalytic Dialogues*, **14**, 605–634.

Wong, E. C., Beutler, L. E. & Zane, N. W. (2007) Using mediators and moderators to test assumptions underlying culturally sensitive therapies: an exploratory example. *Cultural Diversity and Ethnic Minority Psychology*, **13**, 169–177.

CHAPTER 6

Can psychotherapeutic interventions overcome epistemic difference?

Francisco José Eiroa-Orosa and Maria José Fernandez-Gomez

Psychotherapy, indeed the very notion of mental illness and its treatment, are predicated on a modernist epistemic paradigm (Kvale, 1992; Doucet *et al*, 2010). Modernism became the dominant epistemic paradigm in the Western world in the 17th century, when empiricism and reason replaced the idea of direct revelation from God as a way to approach the truth. Modernism in psychotherapy implies a vision of a practitioner who is value-free, objective and unbiased. Postmodernism appeared in the 20th century and questions the very notion of objective truth. Its influence in psychotherapy involves the therapist's awareness of operating from within specific language and sociohistorical frameworks (Lyddon & Weill, 1997).

Kelly (1955) noted that patients try to understand what is going on in their lives in much the same way as scientists try to develop hypotheses about the world; patients have constructions of their reality as scientists have theories. If we understand the psychotherapeutic process as one of scientific interchange and as a form of knowledge generation, we may understand that therapists and patients adopt different roles with differing expectations, depending on the epistemic paradigm they embrace (independently of the awareness they have of it).

The German word *Weltanschauung* (world view) has been extensively used in psychology to refer to sets of assumptions that people use to understand and describe their lived experience of reality. Koltko-Rivera (2004) defines world view as 'a set of beliefs that includes limiting statements and assumptions regarding what exists and what does not (either in actuality, or in principle), what objects or experiences are good or bad, and what objectives, behaviors, and relationships are desirable or undesirable'.

We define epistemic mismatch in psychotherapy or counselling as a phenomenon that would occur when the epistemic vision of therapist and patient belong to different paradigms. This phenomenon may happen in the meeting between people of different cultures whose epistemic views are incompatible (Owusu-Bempah, 2004). A common scenario would be an encounter between a modernist therapist and a patient whose world views collide with rationalism, who relies on mysticism to explain the world. A similar mismatch might occur when a therapist from a more individualistic culture (governed by autonomy or self-determination) tries to understand a patient from a communitarian culture, in which a healthy person is seen as one who is deeply embedded in the community, and self is defined by mutual roles and relationships. Epistemic mismatch can hamper the establishment of a good therapeutic alliance and lead to therapeutic objectives that are incompatible with the patient's way of being in the world. It might also promote a relationship based on intellectual hierarchy rather than collaboration.

An older line of research indicates that the contrast of values in the patient–therapist dyad plays an important role (Pepinsky & Karst, 1964; Beutler, 1981). Although some studies have demonstrated that patients show greater improvement if their therapist shares moderately similar values (Kelly & Strupp, 1992), value convergence in therapy has been associated with the therapist's rating of improvement, but not with the patient's rating (Kelly, 1990).

But how can therapists deal with the problem of objectivity? Husserl was one of the first to introduce the constitution of objectivity in the study of consciousness, although still from a modernist paradigm (Drummond, 1988). According to Husserl's phenomenology, knowledge of essences – how things really are – would be possible only by bracketing all previous assumptions about the existence of an external world (Husserl, 1913). Heidegger (1927) addressed the impossibility of disregarding previous knowledge; Gadamer (1960) went into this idea in depth, arguing that people have an 'historically effected consciousness' (*wirkungsgeschichtliches Bewußtsein*), by which he means that past experience circumscribes future experience. Along the same lines, Kelly (1990) stressed that therapists do not remain value-free even when they intend to do so. This being the case, therapists' disclosure of their world views to patients could be useful as a means of avoiding a hidden clash of paradigms. Although this issue is complex, Henretty & Levitt (2010) suggest that culture may determine the levels of permitted therapist self-disclosure.

The awareness of subjectivity has been brought into clinical practice in different ways, for example, through constructivism (Kelly, 1955), cognitive narrative psychotherapy (Gonçalves, 1994), constructionist/systemic therapy (Real, 1990), and intersubjective and relational approaches (Mitchell, 2000; Orange *et al*, 2001; Yonteff, 2002). In the cross-cultural field, Ibrahim & Arredondo (1986) urge counsellors to adopt a culturally pluralistic attitude. They state that this stance does not assume that any universally agreed world view exists or will ever exist. Nevertheless, Mitchell (1993) concludes that an ethical decision-making process is necessary when world views clash.

According to Kirmayer (2007), the goals and methods of therapeutic change must be appropriate to the patient's cultural concept of the person (for example, the individualistic, egocentric concept of the person can be contrasted with more sociocentric, ecocentric or cosmocentric views). Along these lines, Griner & Smith (2006), in their meta-analytic review, found that adaptations designed to be sensitive to many cultural groups are more efficacious than interventions without any cultural adaptations; and that optimal benefit is achieved when the treatment is tailored to specific cultural contexts. Hall (2001) points out that 'ethical guidelines suggest that psychotherapies be modified to become culturally appropriate for ethnic minority persons', but there is no empirical support for the efficacy of culturally sensitive psychotherapy.

Orientations such as Morita therapy, a Japanese method of treating neurosis (Kora, 1965), and NTU (pronounced 'in-too') therapy, which is based on the core principles of ancient African and Afrocentric world views (Phillips, 1990), use an ethnocentric approach emphasising the critical role that ethnic/racial identity may play in conceptions of mental illness and the process of psychotherapy.

It is unlikely that there is a suitable approach for all patients. In some cases, epistemic differences are an insuperable difficulty. However, in other cases, initial divergence can be transformed into a mutual convergence that is enriching for both patient and therapist. Various cultural, socioeconomic and clinical factors may mediate the appropriateness of a different approach to each case, but often there is no option to choose between different approaches, as access of ethnic minorities to psychotherapy is itself not optimal. We hope that this reflection will help therapists facing the challenge of working with patients whose epistemic views differ from theirs to transform difficulties into mutual enrichment, whether they decide to accept the challenge or decide that a culture-specific approach would better help their clients.

References

Beutler, L. E. (1981) Convergence in counseling and psychotherapy: a current look. *Clinical Psychology Review*, **1**, 79–101.

Doucet, S. A., Letourneau, N. L. & Stoppard, J. M. (2010) Contemporary paradigms for research related to women's mental health. *Health Care for Women International*, **31**, 296–312.

Drummond, J. J. (1988) Modernism and postmodernism: Bernstein or Husserl? *Review of Metaphysics*, **42**, 275–300.

Gadamer, H. G. (1960) *Wahrheit und Methode: Grundzüge einer philosophischen Hermeneutik* [*Truth and Method: Outlines of a Philosophical Hermeneutics*]. J. C. B. Mohr.

Gonçalves, O. F. (1994) Cognitive narrative psychotherapy: the hermeneutic construction of alternative meanings. *Journal of Cognitive Psychotherapy*, **8**, 105–125.

Griner, D., & Smith, T. B. (2006) Culturally adapted mental health interventions: a meta-analytic review. *Psychotherapy: Theory, Research, Practice, Training*, **43**, 531–548.

Hall, G. C. N. (2001) Psychotherapy research with ethnic minorities: empirical, ethical, and conceptual issues. *Journal of Consulting and Clinical Psychology*, **69**, 502–510.

Heidegger, M. (1927) *Sein und Zeit. Gesamtausgabe, Abt. 2* [*Being and Time. Collected Works, Vol. 2*]. Max Niemeyer Verlag.

Henretty, J. R. & Levitt, H. M. (2010) The role of therapist self-disclosure in psychotherapy: a qualitative review. *Clinical Psychology Review*, **30**, 63–77.

Husserl, E. (1913) *Ideen zu einer reinen Phänomenologie und phänomenologischen Philosophie. Erstes Buch: Allgemeine Einführung in die reine Phänomenologie*. Reprinted (1998) as *Ideas Pertaining to a Pure Phenomenology and to a Phenomenological Philosophy: First Book* (trans. F. Kersten). Kluwer Academic.

Ibrahim, F. A. & Arredondo, P. M. (1986) Ethical standards for cross-cultural counseling: preparation, practice, assessment, and research. *Journal of Counseling & Development*, **64**, 349–351.

Kelly, G. A. (1955) *The Psychology of Personal Constructs*. W. W. Norton.

Kelly, T. A. (1990) The role of values in psychotherapy: a critical review of process and outcome effects. *Clinical Psychology Review*, **10**, 171–186.

Kelly, T. A. & Strupp, H. H. (1992) Patient and therapist values in psychotherapy: perceived changes, assimilation, similarity, and outcome. *Journal of Consulting and Clinical Psychology*, **60**, 34–40.

Kirmayer, L. J. (2007) Psychotherapy and the cultural concept of the person. *Transcultural Psychiatry*, **44**, 232–257.

Koltko-Rivera, M. E. (2004) The psychology of worldviews. *Review of General Psychology*, **8**, 3–58.

Kora, T. (1965) Morita therapy. *International Journal of Psychiatry*, **1**, 611–645.

Kvale, S. (1992) Postmodern psychology: a contradiction in terms? In *Psychology and Postmodernism* (ed. S. Kvale), pp. 31–57. Sage.

Lyddon, W. & Weill, R. (1997) Cognitive psychotherapy and postmodernism: emerging themes and challenges. *Journal of Cognitive Psychotherapy*, **11**, 75–91.

Mitchell, D. L. (1993) When the values of clients and counsellors clash: some conceptual and ethical propositions. *Canadian Journal of Counselling and Psychotherapy*, **27**, 203–211.

Mitchell, S. A. (2000) *Relationality: From Attachment to Intersubjectivity*. Analytic Press.

Orange, D. M., Atwood, G. E. & Stolorow, R. D. (2001) *Working Intersubjectively: Contextualism in Psychoanalytic Practice*. Analytic Press.

Owusu-Bempah, K. (2004) Cultural values and community support systems: libertarianism versus communitarianism. *IUC Journal of Social Work Theory & Practice*, **(8)** (http://www.bemidjistate.edu/academics/publications/social_work_journal/issue08/articles/1_Cultural_Values.htm).

Pepinsky, H. B. & Karst, T. O. (1964) Convergence: a phenomenon in counseling and in psychotherapy. *American Psychologist*, **19**, 333–338.

Phillips, F. B. (1990) NTU psychotherapy: an Afrocentric approach. *Journal of Black Psychology*, **17**, 55–74.

Real, T. (1990) The therapeutic use of self in constructionist/systemic therapy. *Family Process*, **29**, 255–272.

Yonteff, G. (2002) The relational attitude in Gestalt therapy theory and practice. *International Gestalt Journal*, **25**, 15–34.

CHAPTER 7

On the role of culture and difference in evaluation, assessment and diagnosis

Adil Qureshi

Culture and difference are considered to have a potentially enormous impact on diagnosis and assessment of mental health and illness, to the extent that some investigators believe that the elevated rates of psychiatric illness in African–Caribbeans in the UK and Holland may be at least in part a function diagnostic error (Hickling *et al*, 1999; Mulder *et al*, 2006; Singh, 2009). Disparities in healthcare can arise from the effect of cultural and racial differences on interactions between patients and mental health services (Smedley *et al*, 2002; Gregg & Saha, 2006). The former has to do with differences in the explanation and expression of mental distress, and treatment expectations and adherence, whereas the latter has to do with noticing differential treatment of individuals on the basis of an arbitrary demographic characteristic (Qureshi *et al*, 2008).

Culture

Culture influences psychiatric diagnosis, especially where there are cultural differences. Psychiatric diagnosis as represented in the Diagnostic and Statistical Manual of Mental Disorders (DSM) and International Classification of Diseases (ICD) systems is predicated on a derived etic or universalist perspective. This holds that mental disorders are real disease entities that exist independent of culture and context, although there are cultural variations in both their expression and explanation, as well as in what is deemed normative and functional (American Psychiatric Association, 1994; Bowers, 1998; Mezzich *et al*, 1999; Kirmayer, 2001). This accommodation of cultural variability, however, is challenging in that the diagnostic systems delimit symptomatology for particular disorders; despite the nod to cultural particularities, in terms of both what constitutes a symptom and how the symptom is related to the disorder, this does not allow for much deviation from Western norms.

The relationship between behaviour, symptom and disorder is complex and rather murky. A particular symptom of a particular disorder in one culture may be normative and functional in another. What is symptomatic of a particular mental disorder according to the DSM system may be symptomatic of a different disorder in another diagnostic system or culture. This is often asserted but rarely supported for culture-bound syndromes. Some symptoms may be indicative of nothing in particular in diagnostic terms. The overall argument is that culture circumscribes, at a very minimum, both expression and explanation of mental distress, and thus the application of standardised diagnostic criteria without taking culture into consideration can result in serious diagnostic error. How can this be?

Culture, mutuality and diagnosis

Diagnosis depends, in part, on the interaction between the clinician and the client. The notion of mutuality holds that the clinician and client affect each other. Thus, the symptoms that a client presents and how they are presented will in part be a function of the relationship with the specific clinician at hand. The clinical gaze is filtered through the particular world view or cosmovision of the latter (Altman, 1999). The interaction between the two is further affected by distinct communication styles at both verbal and non-verbal levels (Qureshi & Collazos, 2011).

Psychometric assessment

Psychometric assessment is predicated on the notion that the construct being measured, be it a mental disorder, a personality attribute or even a specific symptom, is a universally present entity. Consequently, the instrument used has equivalence across cultures and what is measured is a function of the entity in question rather than error or an artefact of cultural difference (Chen, 2008; Byrne *et al*, 2009). Anne Anastasi, expert on psychological testing, noted that 'No test is – or should be – culture-free, because human behavior is not culture-free' (Anastasi, 1989). The implication is that most instruments are plagued with bias, related not only to the construct in question but also to the means by which the information is obtained (method bias) or even the sampling procedures used (van de Vijver & Tanzer, 2004).

Racial/ethnic difference

Race is a highly contested construct, to the extent that in the literature one can find everything from race-based approaches to mental health (Carter, 1995; Metzl, 2009; Fernando, 2010) to calls for rejection of the term in favour of 'ethnicity' in an attempt to avoid the biological determinism often associated with the race construct (American Anthropological Association, 1998). At the same time, 'ethnicity' would appear to invoke some 'cultural' characteristic that is of relevance to the client, whereas 'race' strictly pertains to the arbitrary classification based on the clinician's perception of the client's appearance, generally influenced by contemporary and historical racial (and ethnic) stereotypes.

There is a substantial body of literature that indicates that race influences the reading of symptoms (Bhui *et al*, 2005); African Americans are diagnosed with schizophrenia at a much higher rate than Whites, but with affective disorders at a much lower rate (Strakowski *et al*, 1996; Minsky *et al*, 2003; West *et al*, 2006). The notion of putative psychotic symptoms (Vega *et al*, 2006) refers to ambiguous symptoms that are differentially interpreted according to the race of the patient. In a related vein, race appears to influence psychiatric treatment as well, with people from Black and minority ethnic groups being prescribed fewer atypical antipsychotics (Daumit *et al*, 2003) and subject to more compulsory admissions (Morgan *et al*, 2005; Mulder *et al*, 2006; Ali *et al*, 2007).

The variation in diagnosis, admissions and the like can be understood to be a function of racism (Littlewood, 1992; Abreu, 1999; Ali, 2004). The racism at issue here is not necessarily the more standard overt or explicit racism, but rather what is known as unconscious, modern or aversive racism (Dovidio, 2001; Dovidio *et al*, 2002). This refers to implicit racist behaviour that is beyond conscious control: the clinician more than likely considers himself or herself to be anti-racist, yet, as the research and service evidence suggest, clinicians' responses to Black people are more negative than to White people (Dovidio *et al*, 2008). How can this be explained, without invoking some influence determined by race (or something closely related to it)? Ultimately, these aggregate patterns are a product of interactions at the individual level, influenced by organising structures in services and professional practice.

Recent advances in the neurosciences support notions from both philosophy and psychology which suggest not only that our experience of others is predicated on previous experiences – we never see things as they really are – but also that our very presence affects the behaviour of others (Rorty, 1981; Mitchell, 2000; Han & Northoff, 2008). How a clinician experiences – and affects – culturally and racially different patients can be considerable, and has an impact on psychiatric assessment and diagnosis.

References

Abreu, J. M. (1999) Conscious and nonconscious African American stereotypes: impact on first impression and diagnostic ratings by therapists. *Journal of Consulting and Clinical Psychology*, **67**, 387–393.

Ali, A. (2004) The intersection of racism and sexism in psychiatric diagnosis. In *Bias in Psychiatric Diagnosis* (eds P. J. Caplan & L. Cosgrove), pp. 71–75. Jason Aronson.

Ali, S., Dearman, S. P. & McWilliam, C. (2007) Are Asians at greater risk of compulsory psychiatric admission than Caucasians in the acute general adult setting? *Medicine, Science and the Law*, **47**, 311–314.

Altman, N. (1999) Psychoanalytic perspective on clinical work in the inner city. In *Psychoanalytic Therapy as Health Care: Effectiveness and Economics in the 21st Century* (eds H. Kaley, M. N. Eagle & D. L. Wolitzky), pp. 257–271. Analytic Press.

American Anthropological Association (1998) *American Anthropological Association Statement on "Race"*. American Anthropological Association (http://www.aaanet.org/stmts/racepp.htm).

American Psychiatric Association (1994) *Diagnostic and Statistical Manual of Mental Disorders (4th edn) (DSM-IV)*. American Psychiatric Publishing.

Anastasi, A. (1989) Ability testing in the 1980's and beyond: some major trends. *Public Personnel Management*, **18**, 471–485.

Bhui, K., Stansfeld, S., McKenzie, K., et al (2005) Racial/ethnic discrimination and common mental disorders among workers: findings from the EMPIRIC Study of Ethnic Minority Groups in the United Kingdom. *American Journal of Public Health*, **95**, 496–501.

Bowers, L. (1998) *The Social Nature of Mental Illness*. Routledge.

Byrne, B. M., Oakland, T., Leong, F. T. L., et al (2009) A critical analysis of cross-cultural research and testing practices: implications for improved education and training in psychology. *Training and Education in Professional Psychology*, **3**, 94–105.

Carter, R. T. (1995) *The Influence of Race and Racial Identity in Psychotherapy: Toward a Racially Inclusive Model*. John Wiley & Sons.

Chen, F. F. (2008) What happens if we compare chopsticks with forks? The impact of making inappropriate comparisons in cross-cultural research. *Journal of Personality and Social Psychology*, **95**, 1005–1018.

Daumit, G. L., Crum, R. M., Guallar, E., et al (2003) Outpatient prescriptions for atypical antipsychotics for African Americans, Hispanics, and Whites in the United States. *Archives of General Psychiatry*, **60**, 121–128.

Dovidio, J. F. (2001) On the nature of contemporary prejudice: the third wave. *Journal of Social Issues*, **57**, 829–849.

Dovidio, J. F., Kawakami, K. & Gaertner, S. L. (2002) Implicit and explicit prejudice and interracial interaction. *Journal Personality and Social Psychology*, **82**, 62–68.

Dovidio, J. F., Penner, L. A., Albrecht, T. L., et al (2008) Disparities and distrust: the implications of psychological processes for understanding racial disparities in health and health care. *Social Science & Medicine*, **67**, 478–486.

Fernando, S. (2010) *Mental Health, Race and Culture* (3rd edn). Palgrave Macmillan.

Gregg, J. & Saha, S. (2006) Losing culture on the way to competence: the use and misuse of culture in medical education. *Academic Medicine*, **81**, 542–547.

Han, S. & Northoff, G. (2008) Culture-sensitive neural substrates of human cognition: a transcultural neuroimaging approach. *Nature Review Neurosciences*, **9**, 646–654.

Hickling, F. W., McKenzie, K., Mullen, R., et al (1999) A Jamaican psychiatrist evaluates diagnoses at a London psychiatric hospital. *British Journal of Psychiatry*, **175**, 283–285.

Kirmayer, L. J. (2001) Cultural variations in the clinical presentation of depression and anxiety: implications for diagnosis and treatment. *Journal of Clinical Psychiatry*, **62** (suppl. 13), 22–28.

Littlewood, R. (1992) Psychiatric diagnosis and racial bias: empirical and interpretative approaches. *Social Science & Medicine*, **34**, 141–149.

Metzl, J. M. (2009) *The Protest Psychosis: How Schizophrenia Became a Black Disease*. Beacon Press.

Mezzich, J. E., Kirmayer, L. J., Kleinman, A., et al (1999) The place of culture in DSM-IV. *Journal of Nervous and Mental Disease*, **187**, 457–464.

Minsky, S., Vega, W., Miskimen, T., et al (2003) Diagnostic patterns in Latino, African American, and European American psychiatric patients. *Archives of General Psychiatry*, **60**, 637–644.

Mitchell, S. A. (2000) *Relationality: From Attachment to Intersubjectivity*. Analytic Press.

Morgan, C., Mallett, R., Hutchinson, G., et al (2005) Pathways to care and ethnicity. 1: Sample characteristics and compulsory admission. Report from the ÆSOP study. *British Journal of Psychiatry*, **186**, 281–289.

Mulder, C. L., Koopmans, G. T. & Selten, J.-P. (2006) Emergency psychiatry, compulsory admissions and clinical presentation among immigrants to The Netherlands. *British Journal of Psychiatry*, **188**, 386–391.

Qureshi, A. & Collazos, F. (2011) The intercultural and interracial therapeutic relationship: challenges and recommendations. *International Review of Psychiatry*, **23**, 10–9.

Qureshi, A., Collazos, F., Ramos, M., *et al* (2008) Cultural competency training in psychiatry. *European Psychiatry*, **23** (suppl. 1), 49–58.

Rorty, R. (1981) *Philosophy and the Mirror of Nature*. Princeton University Press.

Singh, S. P. (2009) Shooting the messenger: the science and politics of ethnicity research. *British Journal of Psychiatry*, **195**, 1–2.

Smedley, B. D., Stith, Y. S. & Nelson, A. R. (eds) (2002) *Unequal Treatment: Confronting Racial and Ethnic Disparities in Healthcare*. National Academies Press.

Strakowski, S. M., Flaum, M., Amador, X., *et al* (1996) Racial differences in the diagnosis of psychosis. *Schizophrenia Research*, **21**, 117–124.

van de Vijver, F. & Tanzer, N. K. (2004) Bias and equivalence in cross-cultural assessment. *Revue européen de psychologie appliquée/European Review of Applied Psychology*, **54**, 119–135.

Vega, W. A., Sribney, W. M., Miskimen, T. M., *et al* (2006) Putative psychotic symptoms in the Mexican American population: prevalence and co-occurrence with psychiatric disorders. *Journal of Nervous and Mental Disease*, **194**, 471–477.

West, J. C., Herbeck, D. M., Bell, C. C., *et al* (2006) Race/ethnicity among psychiatric patients: variations in diagnostic and clinical characteristics reported by practicing clinicians. *Focus*, **4**, 48–56.

World Health Organization (1992) *The ICD-10 Classification of Mental and Behavioural Disorders: Clinical Descriptions and Diagnostic Guidelines*. World Health Organization.

CHAPTER 8

Necessary and sufficient competencies for intercultural work

Hilda-Wara Revollo

'Over and over again it has been necessary to learn the lesson that the observer influences the observed. In the field of mental health, we have not only to reckon with the natural effect of the observers' own bias but we also have to deal with a second variable: the effect of this bias on the patient.'

(Jackson, 1960: pp. 5–6)

Intercultural work has converted into a daily reality the challenges of demographic change taking place all over the world (International Organization for Migration, 2012). Professionals who work in intercultural contexts are inevitably affected by the experiences and perceptions of patients from different cultures, and this can place a strain on their professional role (Smedley *et al*, 2002; Qureshi & Collazos, 2005; de Leon Siantz, 2008; Engebretson *et al*, 2008; Clark, 2009; Blume & Lovato, 2010). Mental healthcare professionals continue to raise questions about the sort of knowledge and skills base that contribute most to effective and sensitive intercultural work (Cunningham *et al*, 2002; Kumagai & Lypson, 2009; Ben-Ari & Strier, 2010; Mian *et al*, 2010):

- What sorts of adjustments should one make to meet the needs of a patient from a different culture?
- Beyond linguistic difficulties, manageable with the participation of a medical interpreter or intercultural mediator (see Chapter 11, this volume), what should the clinician keep in mind in order to adequately attend to the patient?
- How can cultural knowledge be applied effectively rather than get in the way?
- What abilities is it most useful to develop?
- Can they be applied to all patients from the same ethnic group?
- Which attitudes facilitate the creation of a therapeutic space and effectiveness in intercultural work? Should the clinician directly raise the matter of clinician–patient differences (race, ethnicity, etc.), or is it better to wait for the patient to take the initiative?

- How can clinicians develop their cultural competence without losing their personal professional style, which is founded on their own professional and cultural background?

Many institutions have published position statements, teaching materials and literature promoting cultural competence. These include the American Psychiatric Association, the Royal College of Psychiatrists, the American Psychological Association, the Australian Psychological Society, the New Zealand Psychological Society, the Canadian Nurses Association, the National Association of Social Workers and the Association Minkowski. The American Psychological Association (2002) encourages ethical and effective multicultural treatment based on the triad of professional–patient–context, with the objective of facilitating access to high-quality therapy regardless of the patient's ethnicity, race or cultural background (Walls, 2004). A variety of models have proposed different ways of developing clinical cultural competence in mental healthcare (Bell *et al*, 2009; Kumagai & Lypson, 2009; Ben-Ari & Strier, 2010; Mian *et al*, 2010), the majority of which centre on three principal dimensions: cultural knowledge, cultural skills, and attitudes and beliefs (Sue *et al*, 1996; Sodowsky *et al*, 1997; Rodolfa *et al*, 2005).

Cultural knowledge and skills

Cultural knowledge encompasses many areas: the patient's culture, world view, language, and expectations of psychotherapy and of the therapeutic relationship; the healthcare model in the patient's country of origin; and any other information related to the patient's beliefs and practices that could affect diagnosis, treatment adherence and the therapeutic relationship (Flores, 2000; Qureshi *et al*, 2008; Sue *et al*, 2009). It is important to know what is germane and relevant at a particular moment: cultural knowledge varies from case to case and subculture to subculture, and reflects the context of the clinician as well as that of the patient (Kleinman, 1980; Bar-Yoseph, 2005; Bryson & Hosken, 2005).

Cultural skills generally refer to the ability to intervene in a culturally sensitive and adequate manner (Sue, 2006). This definition would appear to be general and ambiguous in the face of doubt about what constitutes an adequate intervention for a particular patient with a particular problem in a particular context. Training endeavours in cultural competence focus on developing communication skills (Misra-Herbert, 2003; Browning & Waite, 2010), on the therapeutic relationship (Welch, 2003; Comas-Diaz, 2006; Moran, 2006) and on resources for the negotiation and resolution of problems (Pedersen *et al*, 2008; Gertner *et al*, 2010) in intercultural contexts.

Many training initiatives in clinical cultural competence focus on discovering aspects of the cultural awareness and beliefs of the professional that may affect the development of the therapeutic relationship with a patient from a different culture (Roysircar *et al*, 2003; Beach *et al*, 2005; Roysircar, 2005; Hayes, 2008; Erickson Cornish *et al*, 2010; Mian *et al*, 2010), and there is consequently a strong current encouraging experiential learning (Arthur & Achenbach, 2002; Kim & Lyons, 2003).

There is a lack of awareness among clinicians of their tendency towards bias and of the interplay of culture in intercultural work, and this may be indicated by more overt clinically negligent practice, or just difficulties in the therapeutic relationship and process (Smedley *et al*, 2002; Kirmayer, 2003; Clark, 2009; Sue *et al*, 2009; Blume & Lovato, 2010; Trimble, 2010). All too often in intercultural clinical encounters, the clinician fails to really listen to the patient's demands and needs (Kaplan-Myrth, 2007; Browning & Waite, 2010) and both clinician and patient avoid attending to differences in cultural interpretive filters (Roysircar *et al*, 2003; Bernal & Sáez-Santiago, 2006; Williams, 2006; Bennegadi, 2008; Papadopoulos *et al*, 2008).

Introspection and cultural and racial self-awareness, along with regular supervision and keeping abreast of new developments, continue to be the most recommended practices to avoid problems in clinical contacts (Arredondo & Arciniega, 2001; Smedley *et al*, 2002; Arredondo & Toporek, 2004; Sanchez-Hucles & Jones, 2005; Sue *et al*, 2007; Erickson Cornish *et al*, 2010).

Individual and group supervision, accompanied by the humility necessary to participate in the process of identifying one's cultural and racial transference, are all helpful for intercultural work (Tervalon & Murray-Garcia, 1998; Estrada *et al*, 2004; Haans *et al*, 2007; Haans, 2008; Leavitt, 2010). The process of self-observation requires an ongoing commitment (Stoltenberg, 2005; Sue, 2006) for clinicians to deal with their own cultural beliefs and values that are present in the therapeutic relationship, and that come to the fore during the process of developing cultural sensitivity (Beach *et al*, 2005; White *et al*, 2006; Karamat Ali, 2007).

Both the professional and the patient bring to the consultation room their own attitudes, values, world views and traditions; these influence the therapeutic relationship, evaluation and treatment (Sue & Zane, 1987; Qureshi & Collazos, 2005; Trimble, 2010). Consciousness of prejudices and cultural interpretive filters can transform these from an impediment into a source of information enabling the development of trust and a therapeutic alliance, and identification of therapy-related issues that the patient brings but that might not be otherwise noticed (Satcher, 2000; Zetzer & Shockley, 2006).

Conclusions

Knowledge about the culture of our patients can be very useful for adjusting to their needs. Nevertheless, it is important to establish whether such knowledge is relevant to a particular patient. This can be accomplished using communication, negotiation and problem-resolution skills to identify the knowledge necessary for diagnosis and for a therapeutic relationship that will facilitate treatment adherence. The tendency to generalise information that one has about a culture, about a specific patient, can result in biases that complicate clinical work. It is important to verify that one's cultural knowledge is indeed applicable in each new case (Cuomo & Hogan, 2010).

The principal theories concerning attitudes and the identification of biases and reactions are particularly concerned with the identification of interpretive filters and prejudices that influence our perception. An attitude of openness and cultural humility benefits the therapeutic alliance and, ultimately, the outcome of treatment. Awareness of cultural filters and cultural styles can contribute to a clinician's capacity to facilitate the therapeutic encounter without a loss of their personal and professional style and cultural integrity. The acceptance and subsequent negotiation of the different ways in which symptoms and their causes are expressed and explained can further benefit dialogue between the clinician and patient (Association of American Medical Colleges, 2010).

References

American Psychological Association (2002) *Guidelines on Multicultural Education, Training, Research, Practice, and Organizational Change for Psychologists.* APA (http://www.apa.org/pi/oema/resources/policy/multicultural-guidelines.aspx).

Arredondo, P. & Arciniega, M. G. (2001) Strategies and techniques for counselor training based on the Multicultural Counseling Competencies. *Journal of Mental Health Counseling*, **29**, 263–274.

Arredondo, P. & Toporek, R. (2004) Multicultural counseling competencies = ethical practice. *Journal of Mental Health Counseling*, **26**, 44–56.

Arthur, N. & Achenbach, K. (2002) Developing multicultural counseling competencies through experiential learning. *Counselor Education and Supervision*, **42**, 2–14.

Association of American Medical Colleges (2010) *Tool for Assessing Cultural Competence Training (TACCT)*. AAMC (https://www.aamc.org/download/54344/data/tacct_pdf.pdf).

Bar-Yoseph, T. L. (2005) *The Bridge: Dialogues across Cultures*. Gestalt Institute Press.

Beach, M. C., Price, E. G., Gary, T. L., *et al* (2005) Cultural competence: a systematic review of health care provider educational interventions. *Medical Care*, **43**, 356–373.

Bell, C. C., Wells, S. J. & Merritt, L. M. (2009) Integrating cultural competency and empirically-based practice in child welfare: a model based on community psychiatry field principles of health. *Children and Youth Services Review*, **31**, 1206–1213.

Ben-Ari, A. & Strier, R. (2010) Rethinking cultural competence: what can we learn from Levinas? *British Journal of Social Work*, **40**, 2155–2167.

Bennegadi, R. (2008) Représentations culturelles de la maladie: les apports de l'anthropologie médicale clinique [Cultural representations of illness: the contribution of clinical medical anthropology]. *Psycho-Oncologie*, **2**, 266–270.

Bernal, G. & Sáez-Santiago, E. (2006) Culturally centered psychosocial interventions. *Journal of Community Psychology*, **32**, 121–132.

Blume, A. W. & Lovato, L. V. (2010) Empowering the disempowered: harm reduction with racial/ethnic minority clients. *Journal of Clinical Psychology*, **66**, 189–200.

Browning, S. & Waite, R. (2010) The gift of listening: JUST listening strategies. *Nursing Forum*, **45**, 150–158.

Bryson, J. & Hosken, C. (2005) What does it mean to be a culturally competent I/O psychologist in New Zealand? *New Zealand Journal of Psychology*, **34**, 69–76.

Clark, P. A. (2009) Prejudice and the medical profession: a five-year update. *Journal of Law and Medical Ethics*, **37**, 118–133.

Comas-Diaz, L. (2006) *Cultural Variation in the Therapeutic Relationship*. American Psychological Association.

Cunningham, P. B., Foster, S. L. & Henggeler, S. W. (2002) The elusive concept of cultural competence. *Children's Services: Social Policy, Research, and Practice*, **5**, 231–243.

Cuomo, A. M. & Hogan, M. F. (2010) *Cultural Competence Strategic Plan 2010–2014*. New York State Office of Mental Health (http://www.omh.ny.gov/omhweb/cultural_competence/CC_StrategicPlan.pdf).

de Leon Siantz, M. L. (2008) Leading change in diversity and cultural competence. *Journal of Professional Nursing*, **24**, 167–171.

Engebretson, J., Mahoney, J. & Carlson, E. D. (2008) Cultural competence in the era of evidence-based practice. *Journal of Professional Nursing*, **24**, 172–178.

Erickson Cornish, J. A., Schreier, B. A., Nadkarni, L. I., *et al* (2010) *Handbook of Multicultural Counseling Competencies*. John Wiley & Sons.

Estrada, D., Wiggins Frame, M. & Braun Williams, C. B. (2004) Cross cultural supervision: guiding the conversation toward race and ethnicity. *Journal of Multicultural Counselling and Development*, **32**, 307–319.

Flores, G. (2000) Culture and the patient–physician relationship: achieving cultural competency in health care. *Journal of Pediatrics*, **136**, 14–23.

Gertner, E. J., Sabino, J. N., Mahady, E., *et al* (2010) Developing a culturally competent health network: a planning framework and guide. *Journal of Healthcare Management*, **55**, 190–204.

Haans, T. (2008) Culturally sensitive supervision by expatriate professionals: basic ingredients. *Intervention*, **6**, 140–146.

Haans, T., Lansen, J. & Ten Brummelhuis, H. (2007) Clinical supervision and culture: a challenge in the treatment of persons traumatized by persecution and violence. In *Voices of Trauma across Cultures: Treatment of Posttraumatic States in Global Perspective* (eds J. Wilson & B. Drozdek), pp. 339–366. Springer.

Hayes, P. (2008) *Addressing Cultural Complexities in Practice: Assessment, Diagnosis, and Therapy*. American Psychological Association Press.

International Organization for Migration (2012) Facts & figures: global estimates and trends. IOM.

Jackson, D. (1960) *The Etiology of Schizophrenia*. Basic Books.

Kaplan-Myrth, N. (2007) Interpreting people as they interpret themselves: narrative in medical anthropology and family medicine. *Canadian Family Physician*, **53**, 1268–1269.

Karamat Ali, R. (2007) Learning to be mindful of difference: teaching systemic skills in cross-cultural encounters. *Journal of Family Therapy*, **29**, 368–372.

Kim, B. S. K. & Lyons, H. Z. (2003) Experiential activities and multicultural counseling competence training. *Journal of Counseling & Development*, **81**, 400–408.

Kirmayer, L. J. (2003) Failures of imagination: the refugee's narrative in psychiatry. *Anthropology & Medicine*, **10**, 167–185.

Kleinman, A. (1980) *Patients and Healers in the Context of Culture: An Exploration of the Borderland between Anthropology, Medicine, and Psychiatry*. University of California Press.

Kumagai, A. K. & Lypson, M. L. (2009) Beyond cultural competence: critical consciousness, social justice, and multicultural education. *Academic Medicine*, **84**, 782–787.

Leavitt, R. L. (2010) *Cultural Competence: A Lifelong Journey to Cultural Proficiency*. SLACK.

Mian, A. I., Al-Mateen, C. S. & Cerda, G. (2010) Training child and adolescent psychiatrists to be culturally competent. *Child and Adolescent Psychiatric Clinics of North America*, **19**, 815–831.

Misra-Herbert, A. D. (2003) Physician cultural competence: cross-cultural communication improves care. *Cleveland Clinic Journal of Medicine*, **70**, 289–303.

Moran, J. C. (ed.) (2006) *Dialogues on Difference: Studies of Diversity in the Therapeutic Relationship*. American Psychological Association.

Papadopoulos, I., Tilki, M. & Ayling, S. (2008) Cultural competence in action for CAMHS: development of a cultural competence assessment tool and training programme. *Contemporary Nurse*, **28**, 129–140.

Pedersen, P. B., Crethar, H. C. & Carlson, J. (2008) *Inclusive Cultural Empathy: Making Relationships Central in Counseling and Psychotherapy*. American Psychological Association.

Qureshi, A. & Collazos, F. (2005) Cultural competence in the mental health treatment of immigrant and ethnic minority clients. *Diversity in Health and Social Care*, **2**, 307–317.

Qureshi, A., Collazos, F., Ramos, M., *et al* (2008) Cultural competency training in psychiatry. *European Psychiatry*, **23** (suppl. 1), 49–58.

Rodolfa, E., Bent, R., Eisman, E., *et al* (2005) A cube model for competency development: implications for psychology educators and regulators. *Professional Psychology: Research and Practice*, **36**, 347–354.

Roysircar, G. (2005) Research in multicultural counseling: client needs and counselor competencies. In *Multicultural Issues in Counseling: New Approaches to Diversity* (ed. C. Lee), pp. 369–387. American Counseling Association.

Roysircar, G., Hubbell, R. & Gard, G. (2003) Multicultural research on counselor and client variables: a relational perspective. In *Handbook of Multicultural Competencies in Counseling and Psychology* (eds D. B. Pope-Davis, H. L. K. Coleman, W. Ming Liu, *et al*), pp. 247–266. Sage.

Sanchez-Hucles, J. & Jones, N. (2005) Breaking the silence around race in training, practice, and research. *Counseling Psychologist*, **33**, 547–558.

Satcher, D. (2000) Mental health: a report of the Surgeon General executive summary. *Professional Psychology: Research and Practice*, **31**, 5–13.

Smedley, B. D., Stith, Y. S. & Nelson, A. R. (eds) (2002) *Unequal Treatment: Confronting Racial and Ethnic Disparities in Healthcare*. National Academies Press.

Sodowsky, G. R., Kuo-Jackson, Y. P. & Loya, G. J. (1997) Outcome of training in the philosophy of assessment: multicultural counseling competencies. In *Multicultural Counseling Competencies: Assessment, Education and Training, and Supervision* (eds D. P. Pope-Davis & H. L. K. Coleman), pp. 3–41. Sage.

Stoltenberg, C. (2005) Enhancing professional competence through developmental approaches to supervision. *American Psychologist*, **60**, 857– 864.

Sue, D. W., Ivey, A. E. & Pederson, P. B. (1996) *Theory of Multicultural Counseling and Therapy*. Brooks/Cole.

Sue, D. W., Capodilupo, C. M., Torino, G. C., *et al* (2007) Racial microaggressions in everyday life: implications for clinical practice. *American Psychologist*, **62**, 271–286.

Sue, S. (2006) Cultural competency: from philosophy to research and practice. *Journal of Community Psychology*, **34**, 237–245.

Sue, S. & Zane, N. (1987) The role of culture and cultural techniques in psychotherapy: a critique and reformulation. *American Psychologist*, **42**, 37–45.

Sue, S., Zane, N., Nagayama Hall, G. C., *et al* (2009) The case for cultural competency in psychotherapeutic interventions. *Annual Review of Psychology*, **60**, 525–548.

Tervalon, M. & Murray-Garcia, J. (1998) Cultural humility versus cultural competence: a critical distinction in defining physician training outcomes in multicultural education. *Journal of Health Care for the Poor and Underserved*, **9**, 117–125.

Trimble, J. E. (2010) Bear spends time in our dreams now: magical thinking and cultural empathy in multicultural counselling theory and practice. *Counselling Psychology Quarterly*, **23**, 241–253.

Walls, G. B. (2004) Toward a critical global psychoanalysis. *Psychoanalytic Dialogues*, **14**, 605–634.

Welch, I. D. (2003) *The Therapeutic Relationship: Listening and Responding in a Multicultural World*. Praeger Publishers/Greenwood Publishing Group.

White, T. M., Gibbons, M. B. & Schamberger, M. (2006) Cultural sensitivity and supportive expressive psychotherapy: an integrative approach to treatment. *American Journal of Psychotherapy*, **60**, 299–316.

Williams, C. C. (2006) The epistemiology of cultural competence. *Families in Society: The Journal of Contemporary Social Services*, **87**, 209–220.

Zetzer, H. A. & Shockley, M. E. (2006) *Build the Field and They Will Come: Multicultural Organizational Development for Mental Health Agencies*. The California Endowment.

CHAPTER 9

On the validity and usefulness of existing Eurocentric diagnostic categories

Hilda-Wara Revollo and Jorge Atala-Delgado

'[I]t is clear that there is no classification of the Universe not being arbitrary and full of conjectures. The reason for this is very simple: we do not know what thing the universe is.'

(Borges, 1993)

The principal mental health diagnostic classifications are found in the International Classification of Diseases (ICD) of the World Health Organization (www.who.int/classifications/icd/en) and the Diagnostic and Statistical Manual of Mental Disorders (DSM) of the American Psychiatric Association (www.psych.org/practice/dsm). The DSM was initially developed to create a common system of nomenclature, and the objective of subsequent iterations was the identification of maximally valid diagnostic criteria according to a specific classificatory system. Both the DSM and the ICD systems (despite the ostensible international focus of the latter) are fundamentally based in European and North American thinking (Kleinman, 1988). Western diagnostic systems can be understood in the way that structural anthropology conceptualises scientific classification: 'classificatory schemes [...] allow the natural and social universe to be grasped as an organized whole' (Levi-Strauss, 1966: p. 135).

As a manner of observing the universe, classifications of mental disorders are necessarily immersed in a culture-specific context, which clearly complicates the possibility of their universal application (Heidegger, 2000). Growing multiculturalism demands questioning of the pertinence of these classification systems in non-Western environments. The consequences of generalising data derived from these systems is itself questionable and requires attention (Beneduce, 2006). Three epistemological positions can be distinguished in relation to the question of the validity and/or usefulness of Western diagnostic systems for individuals from non-Western cultures:

- a universally applicable approach, from which the DSM and ICD criteria were born
- a culture-specific approach, in which diagnostic criteria would be developed relative to each culture

- a classification-free approach, which questions the coherence and justification of diagnostic classifications, Western or otherwise.

Classification as universally applicable

The first approach is the most common and shared by mainstream psychiatry. The DSM represents one of the best known systems for the universalisation of psychiatric entities to other cultures (Kupfer *et al*, 2008; Yeung & Kam, 2008). To respond to cultural diversity, DSM-IV (American Psychiatric Association, 1994) made a number of changes from previous editions, including ethnic considerations in research as discussed in the field studies section, a glossary of culture-bound syndromes, guidelines on the cultural formulation model (see Chapter 10, this volume), and the definition of a mental disorder as a clinically significant behavioural or psychological syndrome or pattern that is not merely an expectable and culturally sanctioned response to a particular event.

The principal alternative to categorisation is a dimensional approach, based on the quantification of attributes, taking into consideration the heterogeneity of clinical cases (American Psychiatric Association, 1994). There is some indication that the new edition of the DSM, DSM-5, will pay more attention to dimensionality and its sensitivity to distinct cultural contexts (Escobar & Vega, 2006; Kraemer, 2007; Zachar & Kendler, 2007; Klein, 2008; Alarcón, 2009; Kamphuis & Noordhof, 2009; Maser *et al*, 2009; Widiger, 2011; Livesley, 2012).

Western diagnostic classification systems have been subject to multiple criticisms, reflections and comments concerning their utility, validity and congruence; many authors have raised questions about their universal validity in the context of different subjective realities (Thakker & Ward, 1998; Wen-Shing, 2006; Alarcón, 2009; Flaskerud, 2010; Hofmann *et al*, 2010; Jacob, 2010; Lewis-Fernández *et al*, 2010). Mezzich *et al* (1999), in describing DSM-IV, labelled the manual a 'cultural document' that inevitably reflects the implicit values of Western society despite presenting itself as 'universal, atheoretical, and hence, culture-free'. The principal criticism of this posture is derived from Kleinman's increasingly used concept of the category fallacy (Kleinman, 1976, 1977). This describes what occurs when a diagnostic category from one culture is applied to people from another culture in which it lacks clinical salience and its relevance has not been established, rendering it incoherent (Kleinman, 1987).

Classification as culture specific

This approach posits that some cultural differences can be so great that it is untenable to apply a classification model based in one culture to another (see Chapter 8, this volume). Kirmayer (2007), despite working from a universally applicable perspective, approaches this question looking at the cultural concepts of the person. He recommends differences in psychotherapeutic treatment depending on whether the self is egocentric, sociocentric, ecocentric or cosmocentric. If Western classifications are predicated on an egocentric self, the degree to which they could be applied to others sorts of selves is questionable.

Given the difficulties, if not the impossibility, of effective application of Western diagnostic models in non-Western societies, some propose the use of culture-specific diagnostic systems such as those of Latin America (Berganza *et al*, 2002) and China (Chinese Psychiatric Association, 2000). Systemic approaches take the position that mental health problems occur in the context of a system (family or otherwise), even if an individual is identified as symptomatic (Watzlawick *et al*, 1974). A circular, non-linear logic, in which there is no specific beginning or end, is favoured over the Cartesian cause–effect model. Culture-specific classification makes sense because of the possible incompatibility of logical systems across cultures. Critics of such an approach hold that different societies and groups have much in common, although they recognise and are sensitive to cultural differences. Furthermore, the culture-specific approach limits clinicians to diagnosing only members of their own cultural group, producing a practically untenable situation in most services, where cultural matching is not possible. Indeed, much therapeutic work does take place cross-culturally.

Classification-free approach

Classification in general, and diagnostic systems specifically, are called into question by those who underscore the difficulties inherent in fitting what appear to be unclassifiable and perhaps incomprehensible behaviours and symptom clusters into predetermined categories (Levi-Strauss, 1966). It is argued that mental health diagnosis and care should be adapted to each new person, situation and so on (Le Gaufey, 2006), to not lose sight of the complexity and richness of the individual patient's characteristics (Andreasen, 2007). The other two positions demonstrate the need and/or utility of their respective classification systems. This third one is predicated on the position that the mere act of categorisation results in reductionism and bias (Szasz, 1961; Martin & Sugarman, 2001; Olesen, 2003).

Concluding thoughts

Taking into account these epistemological positions concerning diagnostic classification in mental health, what do we do when we have a patient from an unfamiliar culture who would appear to fit into an existing diagnostic category? Is their poor response to an apparently indicated treatment indicative of the category fallacy, or is it simply due to a knowledge deficit that psychiatry has yet to fill? Does the use of classifications (diagnostic or otherwise) in and of itself help us provide quality services to our culturally different patients, does it get in our way, or is the real issue one of striving for culturally competent classifications?

In the face of these concerns, we suggest that the following points are taken into consideration:

- Any classification system is predicated on a specific socioeconomic, historical and political context and a concrete cultural filter. Knowing our own position with regard to these factors can help us understand how distortions might arise when systems are applied to patients from other cultures.
- The use of any classification system can make it easier to lose sight of the complexity and richness of the patient and, as a consequence, result in a biased perception based on our own cultural, personal and professional filters (e.g. the biomedical model; the particular healthcare system; epistemologically preferred professional perspectives).
- Biases or poor interpretations are more frequent with patients from cultures and ethnicities with which we are not familiar. To be alert to the cultural knowledge that we have and see to what point it is pertinent to a specific patient is the principal challenge. Flexibility and awareness of both of the interpretive filters in play (that of the patient and that of the clinician) can help considerably.

References

Alarcón, R. D. (2009) Inside the DSM-V process: issues, debates, and reflections. *Psychiatric Times*, **26**, 1.

American Psychiatric Association (1994) *Diagnostic and Statistical Manual of Mental Disorders (4th edn) (DSM-IV)*. American Psychiatric Publishing.

Andreasen, N. C. (2007) DSM and the death of phenomenology in America: an example of unintended consequences. *Schizophrenia Bulletin*, **33**, 108–112.

Beneduce, R. (2006) Enfermedad, persona y saberes de la curación: entre la cultura y la historia [Illness, the person and knowledge of healing: between culture and history]. *Anales de Antropología*, **40**, 1.

Berganza, C. E., Mezzich, J. E. & Jorge, M. R. (2002) Latin American Guide for Psychiatric Diagnosis (GLDP). *Psychopathology*, **35**, 185–190.

Borges, J. L. (1993) The analytical language of John Wilkins. In *Other Inquisitions 1937–1952* (ed. J. F. Solem, trans. L. Graciela Vázquez & R. L. C. Simms), pp. 101–105. University of Texas Press.

Chinese Psychiatric Association (2000) *Chinese Classification of Mental Disorders*. Shandong Science Press.

Escobar, J. I. & Vega, W. A. (2006) Cultural issues and psychiatric diagnosis: providing a general background for considering substance use diagnoses. *Addiction*, **101**, 40–47.

Flaskerud, J. H. (2010) DSM proposed changes. Part I: Criticisms and influences on changes. *Issues in Mental Health Nursing*, **31**, 686–688.

Heidegger, M. (2000) I: The idea of philosophy and the problem of worldview. In *Towards the Definition of Philosophy* (trans. T. Sadler), pp. 1–99. Athlone Press.

Hofmann, S. G., Anu Asnaani, M. A. & Hinton, D. E. (2010) Cultural aspects in social anxiety and social anxiety disorder. *Depression and Anxiety*, **27**, 1117–1127.

Jacob, K. S. (2010) Indian psychiatry and classification of psychiatric disorders. *Indian Journal of Psychiatry*, **52** (suppl. 1), S104–S109.

Kamphuis, J. H. & Noordhof, A. (2009) On categorical diagnoses in DSM-V: cutting dimensions at useful points? *Psychological Assessment*, **21**, 294–301.

Kirmayer, L. J. (2007) Psychotherapy and the cultural concept of the person. *Transcultural Psychiatry*, **44**, 232–257.

Klein, D. N. (2008) Classification of depressive disorders in the DSM-V: proposal for a two-dimension system. *Journal of Abnormal Psychology*, **117**, 552–560.

Kleinman, A. (1976) Concepts and a model for the comparison of medical systems as cultural systems. *Social Science and Medicine*, **12**, 85–93.

Kleinman, A. (1977) Depression, somatization, and the 'new cross-cultural psychiatry'. *Social Science and Medicine*, **11**, 3–10.

Kleinman, A. (1987) Anthropology and psychiatry: the role of culture in cross-cultural research on illness. *British Journal of Psychiatry*, **151**, 447–454.

Kleinman, A. (1988) *Rethinking Psychiatry: From Cultural Category to Personal Experience*. The Free Press.

Kraemer, H. C. (2007) DSM categories and dimensions in clinical and research contexts. *International Journal of Methods in Psychiatric Research*, **16** (suppl. 1), S8–S15.

Kupfer, D., Regier, D. A. & Kuhl, E. A. (2008) On the road to DSM-V and ICD-11. *European Archives of Psychiatry and Clinical Neuroscience*, **258**, 2–6.

Le Gaufey, G. (2006) *Le Pastout De Lacan: Consistance Logique, Conséquences Cliniques [Lacan's 'Pas-tout': Logical Consistency, Clinical Impact]*. EPEL.

Levi-Strauss, C. (1966) *The Savage Mind* (trans. J. Weightman & D. Weightman). University of Chicago Press.

Lewis-Fernández, R., Hinton, D. E., Laria, A. J., et al (2010) Culture and the anxiety disorders: recommendations for DSM-V. *Depression and Anxiety*, **27**, 212–229.

Livesley, W. J. (2012) Disorder in the proposed DSM-5 classification of personality disorders. *Clinical Psychology & Psychotherapy*, **19**, 364–368.

Martin, J. & Sugarman, J. (2001) Interpreting human kinds: beginnings of a hermeneutic psychology. *Theory & Psychology*, **11**, 193–207.

Maser, J. D., Norman, S. B., Zisook, S., et al (2009) Psychiatric nosology is ready for a paradigm shift in DSM-V. *Clinical Psychology: Science and Practice*, **16**, 24–40.

Mezzich, J. E., Kirmayer, L. J., Kleinman, A., et al (1999) The place of culture in DSM-IV. *Journal of Nervous and Mental Disease*, **187**, 457–464.

Olesen, J. (2003) Examination and interpretation in a phenomenological and hermeneutical biopsychosocial holistic perspective. *Nordisk Psykologi*, **55**, 235–264.

Szasz, T. (1961) *The Myth of Mental Illness: Foundations of a Theory of Personal Conduct*. Hoeber-Harper.

Thakker, J. & Ward, T. (1998) Culture and classification: the cross-cultural application of the DSM-IV. *Clinical Psychology Review*, **18**, 501–529.

Watzlawick, P., Weakland, J. H. & Fisch, R. (1974) *Change: Principles of Problem Formation and Problem Resolution*. W. W. Norton.

Wen-Shing, T. (2006) From peculiar psychiatric disorders through culture-bound syndromes to culture-related specific syndromes. *Transcultural Psychiatry*, **43**, 554–576.

Widiger, T. A. (2011) The DSM-5 dimensional model of personality disorder: rationale and empirical support. *Journal of Personality Disorders*, **25**, 222–234.

Yeung, A. & Kam, R. (2008) Ethical and cultural considerations in delivering psychiatric diagnosis: reconciling the gap using MDD diagnosis delivery in less-acculturated Chinese patients. *Transcultural Psychiatry*, **45**, 531–552.

Zachar, P. & Kendler, K. S. (2007) Psychiatric disorders: a conceptual taxonomy. *American Journal of Psychiatry*, **164**, 557–565.

CHAPTER 10

Benefits and limitations of the cultural formulation in intercultural work

Francisco Collazos, Marcos González and Adil Qureshi

In 1991, the US National Institute of Mental Health supported the creation of the Group on Culture and Diagnosis. The main goal of this group was to advise the DSM-IV Task Force on how to make culture more central to DSM-IV (Mezzich, 1995). The Group even suggested the inclusion of a sixth axis devoted to cultural issues. This ambitious proposal had to be abandoned because of the strong criticisms received but, among the few suggestions finally accepted, the 'cultural formulation' was probably the most significant (Mezzich *et al*, 1999).

The cultural formulation is an operationalisation for clinicians of the process of cultural analysis as it relates to the clinical encounter that can be performed as part of the evaluation of every patient. From the outset, one of its specific aims was to provide a mechanism that would facilitate the application of a cultural perspective to the process of clinical interviewing and diagnostic formulation in psychiatry (Lewis-Fernàndez, 1996). The cultural formulation was meant to supplement the multi-axial diagnostic assessment and to address difficulties that may be encountered in applying DSM-IV criteria in a multicultural environment. The DSM cultural formulation consists of five components:

- assessing cultural identity
- cultural explanations of the illness
- cultural factors related to the psychosocial environment and levels of functioning
- cultural elements of the clinician–patient relationship
- the overall influence of culture on diagnosis and care.

As explained by the Committee on Cultural Psychiatry of the Group for the Advancement of Psychiatry, the specific definitions, causal role and interrelations of constructs such as culture, immigration, ethnic identity and so forth are difficult to delineate, to the extent that these constructs are confounded or lost (Committee on Cultural Psychiatry, 2002). In addition, as some authors have pointed out (Alarcón, 1995; Bäärnhielm

& Rosso, 2009), a key challenge in cultural psychiatry is the management of the nomothetic *v.* the idiographic. The cultural formulation seeks to aid clinicians in combining the more idiographic perspective of psychiatry and the DSM with the more nomothetic (Bäärnhielm & Rosso, 2009).

Benefits

In the DSM cultural formulation, culture is conceptualised as heterogeneous, embodied and continuous. Culture is always dynamic, polyphonic and multifaceted. These cognitive perspectives are not complete, not immutable; culture is communication and interaction, and is embodied in several ways. Personal meanings are linked with collective meanings and always interacting (Borra, 2008). Culture is as much a process as an entity (Greenfield, 1997). Attempts to freeze culture into a set of generalised value orientations or behaviours will continually misrepresent what culture is. Culture is a dynamic and creative process, some aspects of which are shared by large groups of individuals as a result of particular life circumstances and histories (López & Guarnaccia, 2000).

To provide a comprehensive meaning of the lived experience of culture, the cultural formulation is based on the patient's narrative, in much the same way as in psychodynamic approaches and in contrast to the categorical models of multi-axial classifications. The narrative model offers evident advantages from a practical point of view. First, it allows for greater flexibility and is easier to carry out when it comes to capturing different characteristics from a large variety of patients. Second, it captures the subjectivity of the patient, which helps the clinician form a more humane and individualised clinical picture of the individual (Lewis-Fernàndez, 1996)

Limitations

The literature contains few case histories predicated on the cultural formulation model, and the narrative style is absent from most of them. López & Guarnaccia (2000) underscore this tension concerning how the construct of culture is used in assessment, that is, to what extent it is given explanatory (nomothetic) power, in the process of which the specifics of the particular patient are lost (Lu *et al*, 1995). This can be seen in case histories in which general cultural information is provided that may or may not be germane to the patient being discussed, and in which the cultural formulation runs the risk of thematising the cultural perspective, losing the patient and their particular perspective in the process. To that end, a return to the original spirit of the cultural formulation would be beneficial, that is, a return to the patient's narrative (Lewis-Fernàndez & Diaz, 2002). A review of many of the cases published in the journal *Culture, Medicine and*

Psychiatry suggests that a further step is needed to bridge the gap between the culture of the individual and the individuals themselves.

A number of reasons might account for the low use of the cultural formulation. In part, it could be related to its format and applicability: a full cultural formulation takes time – time that simply is not available in standard clinical practice. Furthermore, its implementation might become repetitive if some data have already been gathered in the regular clinical history.

A number of weaknesses have been pointed out in the DSM-IV cultural formulation, and these should be attended to in future versions. For example, the presence of an interpreter or the patient's preferences regarding the therapist's gender and nationality can influence the interaction, as can previous experiences of discrimination in healthcare or of barriers to healthcare resources; the patient's subculture may be relevant, as might their concepts of their own culture and the host culture. Bäärnhielm & Rosso (2009) and Kirmayer *et al* (2008) highlight the importance of including questions about migration, acculturation and religion in the outline of the cultural formulation.

Various authors have created extended versions of the DSM cultural formulation, to facilitate implementation of the instrument in clinical practice. For example, the McGill-JGH Cultural Consultation Service has developed two extended versions based on the DSM-IV outline (www. mcgill.ca/iccc/resources/cf), and a team in The Netherlands has used it as the basis of a Dutch-language interview (Rohlof & Ghane, 2003), which has been translated into English (Rohlof *et al*, 2008). Another team has adapted the DSM formulation to the Swedish context (Bäärnhielm *et al*, 2007; Bäärnhielm & Rosso, 2009).

Notwithstanding its limitations, a clinician who consistently applies the DSM-IV's cultural formulation will surely be more effective than a clinician who remains ignorant of the powerful influence that culture and ethnicity have on both patient and doctor (López & Guarnaccia, 2000; Graham Shaffer & Steiner, 2006)

References

Alarcón, R. D. (1995) Culture and psychiatric diagnosis: impact on DSM-IV and ICD-10. *Psychiatric Clinics of North America*, **18**, 449–465.

Bäärnhielm, S. & Rosso, M. S. (2009) The Cultural Formulation: a model to combine nosology and patients' life context in psychiatric diagnostic practice. *Transcultural Psychiatry*, **46**, 406–428.

Bäärnhielm, S., Rosso, M. S. & Pattyi L. (2007) *Culture, Context and Psychiatric Diagnosis: Interview Manual for the Outline for a Cultural Formulation in DSM-IV* (trans. S. Wicks & S. Bäärnhielm). Transcultural Centre, Stockholm County Council (http://www.slso.sll.se/upload/Transkulturellt%20Centrum/SB%202009-04-14%20swws.pdf).

Borra, R. (2008) Working with the cultural formulation in therapy. *European Psychiatry*, **23** (suppl. 1), 43–48.

Committee on Cultural Psychiatry (2002) *Cultural Assessment in Clinical Psychiatry.* American Psychiatric Publishing.

Graham Shaffer, T. & Steiner, H. (2006) An application of DSM-IV's outline for cultural formulation: understanding conduct disorder in Latino adolescents. *Aggression and Violent Behavior*, **11**, 655–663.

Greenfield, P. M. (1997) Culture as process: empirical methods for cultural psychology. In *Handbook of Cross-Cultural Psychology. Vol. 1 Theory and Method* (eds J. W. Berry, Y. H. Poortinga & J. Pandey), pp. 301–346. Allyn & Bacon.

Kirmayer, L. J., Thombs, B. D., Jurcik, T., *et al* (2008) Use of an expanded version of the DSM-IV outline for cultural formulation on a cultural consultation service. *Psychiatric Services*, **59**, 683–686.

Lewis-Fernàndez, R. (1996) Cultural formulation of psychiatric diagnosis. *Culture, Medicine and Psychiatry*, **20**, 133–144.

Lewis-Fernàndez, R. & Diaz, N. (2002) The cultural formulation: a method for assessing cultural factors affecting the clinical encounter. *Psychiatric Quarterly*, **73**, 271–295.

López, S. R. & Guarnaccia, P. J. (2000) Cultural psychopathology: uncovering the social world of mental illness. *Annual Review of Psychology*, **51**, 571–598.

Lu, F. G., Lim, R. & Mezzich, J. E. (1995) Issues in the assessment and diagnosis of culturally diverse individuals. In *Review of Psychiatry* (eds J. Oldham & M. Riba), pp. 477–510. American Psychiatric Press.

Mezzich, J. E. (1995) Cultural formulation and comprehensive diagnosis: clinical and research perspectives. *Psychiatric Clinics of North America*, **18**, 649–657.

Mezzich, J. E., Kirmayer, L. J., Kleinman, A., *et al* (1999) The place of culture in DSM-IV. *Journal of Nervous and Mental Disease*, **187**, 457–464.

Rohlof, J. F. & Ghane, S. (2003) Het culturele interview [The cultural interview]. In *Cultuursensitief werken met DSM-IV [Culture Sensitive Work with DSM-IV]* (eds R. van Dijk & N. Sönmez), pp. 49–52. Mikado.

Rohlof, H., Loevy, N., Sassen, L., *et al* (2008) *The Cultural Formulation Interview: English version.* H. Rohlof (http://www.rohlof.nl/culturalint.htm).

CHAPTER 11

Barriers to the intercultural therapeutic relationship and how to overcome them

Adil Qureshi and Rachel Tribe

A considerable body of research shows that ethnic minorities and immigrants have lower levels of health service use relative to White or mainstream populations (Institute of Medicine, 2002), and once entering into treatment, have poorer adherence and end it sooner. These results are in part due to barriers related to access to mental health services, poor awareness of mental health services and stigma surrounding their use, lack of services in the patient's mother tongue, cultural insensitivity (Sue, 2003), distrust of service providers (Watkins *et al*, 1989) and problems in the therapeutic relationship (Griffith, 1977; Welch, 2003; Qureshi, 2005; Comas-Diaz, 2006; Qureshi & Collazos, 2011).

Some of these barriers lie beyond the purview of the busy mental health professional. The therapeutic relationship, however, is not only well within the control of the clinician, it is also one of the strongest predictors of positive therapeutic outcome (Horvath & Symonds, 1991; Jennings & Skovholt, 1999; Martin *et al*, 2000; Cruz & Pincus, 2002). The barriers can be understood to be related to sociorace and racism and cultural difference (Gregg & Saha, 2006). The impact of the last derives from the cultural encapsulation of the clinician (Wrenn, 1985), in which the clinician operates from the perspective of pig-headed ethnocentrism (as differentiated from quotidian ethnocentrism in which the clinician is aware that they experience the world from their own cultural perspective) (Rorty, 1987), assuming that their own take on reality is not only correct but also superior to that of the ethnic other. The power differential inherent in the clinical context (Rose, 1998), which can be exacerbated by institutional racism and the challenges inherent in immigration (Walls, 2004), can negatively affect the therapeutic relationship in various ways.

Intercultural communication

Communication style, both verbal and non-verbal, is culturally circumscribed (Singh *et al*, 1998; Morales *et al*, 1999; McDonagh, 2000; Skelton *et al*,

2001; Ulrey & Amason, 2001; Van Wieringen *et al*, 2002; Kapoor *et al*, 2003; Misra-Herbert, 2003). Normal and adequate communication is a function of cultural context. In the clinical encounter, too little or too much expression of emotion (either flat affect or lability), for example, is considered to be symptomatic. Yet it is reasonably well established that norms for the expression of emotion are by no means universal (Markus & Kitayama, 1991; Jenkins, 1996). Communication is increasingly understood to be dialogical and mutual, that is, each participant affects the other (Orange *et al*, 2001; Skelton *et al*, 2001).

Cultural values

Differences in cultural values (Hall & Hall, 1990; Carter, 1991; Hofstede, 1991; Sue & Sue, 1999; Li & Kim, 2004; Bhui & Dinos, 2008), which act as our interpretive filters or the basis of how we make sense of and interact with the world, can negatively affect the therapeutic encounter. In a nutshell, the suggestion is that the therapeutic endeavour suffers when clinician and patient operate from within different paradigms: in effect, they experience, express (Mezzich *et al*, 1999; Barrio *et al*, 2003) and explain (Patel, 1995; Bhui & Bhugra, 2002; McCabe & Priebe, 2004) reality using different parameters.

Given that we automatically interpret others through our own cultural filters, if we do not take these differences into consideration, all too easily, as is the case with different communication styles and cultural values, we may view others as deficient, rude, pathological, non-normative, when in fact they are behaving in a manner syntonic with their own culture. We do not truly 'see' the other person, and they react accordingly (and indeed may not 'see' us either), and negative interactions result.

Racism

Racism has been defined as the combination of prejudice and power (Carter, 2007), and in the clinical context it usually operates at the level of aversive or unconscious racism (Kovel, 1984; Whaley, 1998; Dovidio, 2001; Altman, 2002; Quillian, 2008). The clinician is likely to be overtly or explicitly non-racist if not anti-racist, yet their implicit behaviour belies at the very minimum an own-group preference (Banaji *et al*, 1997; Greenwald *et al*, 2009). The clinician will not be aware of this – they will be convinced that they are behaving in an exemplary manner. The patient, however, may be alert to the implicitly racist or racialist behaviour of the clinician, and this can have a direct impact on the development of the therapeutic relationship, particularly as it can all too easily give rise to serious mistrust of the clinician's skill and concern (Watkins, *et al*, 1989; Whaley, 2001). A revealing experiment is to try the Implicit Association Test, which is designed to demonstrate conscious–unconscious divergences in our attitudes (https://implicit.harvard.edu/implicit).

Countertransference

A number of researchers from around the world have identified racial or cultural transference as the means by which clinicians avoid confronting their own uncomfortable race-related issues, in the process distorting the way they see, and thus engage with, the patient (e.g. Griffith, 1977; Comas-Diaz & Jacobsen, 1991; Blue & Gonzalez, 1992; Yi, 1995; Gorkin, 1996; Holmes, 2001; Altman, 2002). A patient from an ethnic minority can be deracialised by conceiving of them as exotic, as someone who needs to be taken care of by the privileged and dominant group, by denying the reality or pertinence of racism, or indeed by viewing them as a problem. In all of these variations, the person of the patient is in effect ignored in favour of a stereotype, a fantasy that derives from the clinician's past and unconscious avoidance of confronting racial difference in the therapeutic encounter.

Overcoming barriers

Therapist self-awareness

The old adage 'physician, know thyself' should form the foundation of the therapeutic relationship with patients, regardless of their cultural background. This is enshrined in the 'attitudes' dimension of cultural competence (see Chapter 8, this volume) (Arredondo, 1998; Mitchell, 2000; Arthur & Achenbach, 2002; Kim & Lyons, 2003). Indeed, experiential approaches to cultural competency training are popular precisely because they provide a forum in which the clinician can explore and attend to their own issues. This includes exploration of their own ethnic and racial heritage, sexual orientation, gender, age and the like, in as much as own-group attitudes can affect other-group perspectives. It also means exploration of their prejudices, those implicit associations and automatic reactions. However, some commentators suggest that the focus on race and ethnicity is overblown, and what is needed is effective application of generic counselling skills (Patterson, 2004).

Basic training in cultural psychiatry

Awareness of how culture influences the patient's experience, expression and explanation of mental distress as well as their expectations of treatment can be of considerable utility for the clinician as an orienting paradigm. With such awareness – not necessarily in the form of specific knowledge about specific cultures – the clinician can monitor their own reactions and explore the degree to which they are accurate.

Communication skills training

Basic training in intercultural communication specifically and communication in general can be a tremendous help. Experiential training provides specific activities in which the clinician can explore first hand the impact of cultural difference on communication, and have the opportunity to try out different means of overcoming these differences.

Developing flexibility

Taking a flexible approach in which standard practice can be suspended in favour of a more open and accommodating response (within the context of professional boundaries and integrity) can be invaluable. At the very least, it means that many accepted therapeutic 'commandments' can be put into abeyance or reconsidered in light of the interaction with the specific patient.

Supervision

Achievement of self-awareness and exploration of prejudices, transference and interpretive filters are difficult if not impossible to manage alone: it is very hard to see ourselves from anything but our own automatic perspective. To that end, process-oriented multicultural supervision is highly recommended.

References and further reading

Altman, N. (2002) Black and White thinking: a psychoanalyst reconsiders race. *Psychoanalytic Dialogues*, **10**, 589–605.

Arredondo, P. (1998) Integrating multicultural counseling competencies and universal helping conditions in culture-specific contexts. *Counseling Psychologist*, **26**, 592–601.

Arthur, N. & Achenbach, K. (2002) Developing multicultural counseling competencies through experiential learning. *Counselor Education & Supervision*, **42**, 2–14.

Banaji, M. R., Blair, I. V. & Glaser, J. (1997) Environments and unconscious processes. In *The Automaticity of Everyday Life: Advances in Social Cognition* (ed. R. S. Wyer), pp. 63–74. Lawrence Erlbaum Associates.

Barrio, C., Yamada, A., Atuel, H., *et al* (2003) A tri-ethnic examination of symptom expression on the positive and negative syndrome scale in schizophrenia spectrum disorders. *Schizophrenia Research*, **60**, 259–269.

Bhui, K. & Bhugra, D. (2002) Explanatory models for mental distress: implications for clinical practice. *British Journal of Psychiatry*, **181**, 6–7.

Bhui, K. & Dinos, S. (2008) Health beliefs and culture: essential considerations for outcome measurement. *Disease Management and Health Outcomes*, **16**, 411–419.

Blue, H. C. & Gonzalez, C. A. (1992) The meaning of ethnocultural difference: its impact on and use in the psychotherapeutic process. In *Treating Diverse Disorders with Psychotherapy: New Directions for Mental Health Services* (ed. D. Greenfeld), pp. 73–84. Jossey-Bass.

Carter, R. T. (1991) Cultural values: a review of empirical research and implications for counseling. *Journal of Counseling and Development*, **70**, 164–173.

Carter, R. T. (2007) Racism and psychological and emotional injury: recognizing and assessing race-based traumatic stress. *Counseling Psychologist*, **35**, 13–105.

Comas-Diaz, L. (2006) *Cultural Variation in the Therapeutic Relationship*. American Psychological Association.

Comas-Diaz, L. & Jacobsen, F. M. (1991) Ethnocultural transference and countertransference in the therapeutic dyad. *American Journal of Orthopsychiatry*, **61**, 392–402.

Cruz, M. & Pincus, H. A. (2002) Research on the influence that communication in psychiatric has on treatment. *Psychiatric Services*, **53**, 1253–1265.

Dovidio, J. F. (2001) On the nature of contemporary prejudice: the third wave. *Journal of Social Issues*, **57**, 829–849.

Gorkin, M. (1996) Countertransference in cross-cultural psychotherapy. In *Reaching across Boundaries of Culture and Class: Widening the Scope of Psychotherapy* (eds R. M. P. Foster, M. Moskowitz & R. A. Javiev), pp. 159–176. J. Aronson.

Greenwald, A. G., Poehlman, T. A., Uhlmann, E. L., *et al* (2009) Understanding and using the Implicit Association Test: III. Meta-analysis of predictive validity. *Journal of Personality and Social Psychology*, **97**, 17–41.

Gregg, J. & Saha, S. (2006) Losing culture on the way to competence: the use and misuse of culture in medical education. *Academic Medicine*, **81**, 542–547.

Griffith, M. S. (1977) The influences of race on the psychotherapeutic relationship. *Psychiatry*, **40**, 27–40.

Hall, E. T. & Hall, M. R. (1990) *Understanding Cultural Differences*. Intercultural Press.

Hofstede, G. H. (1991) *Cultures and Organizations: Software of the Mind*. McGraw Hill.

Holmes, D. E. (2001) Race and countertransference: two "blind spots" in psychoanalytic perception. In *The Psychoanalytic Century: Freud's Legacy for the Future* (ed. D. E. Scharff), pp. 251–268. Other Press.

Horvath, A. O. & Symonds, B. D. (1991) Relation between working alliance and outcome in psychotherapy: a meta-analysis. *Journal of Counseling and Development*, **38**, 139–149.

Institute of Medicine (2002) *Unequal Treatment: Confronting Racial and Ethnic Disparities in Healthcare*. National Academies Press.

Jenkins, J. H. (1996) Culture, emotion, and psychiatric disorder. In *Medical Anthropology: Contemporary Theory and Method* (eds C. F. Sargent & M. Thomas), pp. 71–87. Praeger.

Jennings, L. & Skovholt, T. M. (1999) The cognitive, emotional, and relational characteristics of master therapists. *Journal of Counseling Psychology*, **46**, 3–11.

Kapoor, S., Hughes, P. C., Baldwin, J. R., *et al* (2003) The relationship of individualism–collectivism and self-construals to communication styles in India and the United States. *International Journal of Intercultural Relations*, **27**, 683–700.

Kim, B. S. K. & Lyons, H. Z. (2003) Experiential activities and multicultural counseling competence training. *Journal of Counseling & Development*, **81**, 400–408.

Kovel, J. (1984) *White Racism: A Psychohistory*. Columbia University Press.

Li, L. C. & Kim, B. S. K. (2004) Effects of counseling style and client adherence to Asian cultural values on counseling process with Asian American college students. *Journal of Counseling Psychology*, **51**, 158–167.

Markus, H. R. & Kitayama, S. (1991) Culture and self: implications for cognition, emotion, and motivation. *Psychological Review*, **98**, 224–253.

Martin, D. J., Garske, J. P. & Davis, M. K. (2000) Relation of therapeutic alliance with outcome and other variables: a meta-analytic review. *Journal of Consulting and Clinical Psychology*, **68**, 438–450.

McCabe, R. & Priebe, S. (2004) Explanatory models of illness schizophrenia: comparison of four ethnic groups. *British Journal of Psychiatry*, **185**, 25–30.

McDonagh, M. S. (2000) Cross-cultural communication and pharmaceutical care. *Drug Topics*, **144**, 95–104.

Mezzich, J. E., Kirmayer, L. J., Kleinman, A., *et al* (1999) The place of culture in DSM-IV. *Journal of Nervous and Mental Disease*, **187**, 457–464.

Misra-Herbert, A. (2003) Physician cultural competence: cross-cultural communication improves care. *Cleveland Clinic Journal of Medicine*, **70**, 289–303.

Mitchell, S. A. (2000) *Relationality: From Attachment to Intersubjectivity*. Analytic Press.

Morales, L. S., Cunningham, W. E., Brown, J. A., *et al* (1999) Are Latinos less satisfied with communication by health care providers? *Journal of General Internal Medicine*, **14**, 409–417.

Orange, D. M., Atwood, G. E. & Stolorow, R. D. (2001) *Working Intersubjectively: Contextualism in Psychoanalytic Practice*. Analytic Press.

Patel, V. (1995) Explanatory models of mental illness in Sub-Saharan Africa. *Social Science and Medicine*, **40**, 1291–1298.

Patterson, C. H. (2004) Do we need multicultural counseling competencies? *Journal of Mental Health Counseling*, **26**, 67–74.

Quillian, L. (2008) Does unconscious racism exist? *Social Psychology Quarterly*, **71**, 6–11.

Qureshi, A. (2005) Dialogical relationship and cultural imagination: a hermeneutic approach to intercultural psychotherapy. *American Journal of Psychotherapy*, **59**, 119–135.

Qureshi, A. & Collazos, F. (2011) The intercultural and interracial therapeutic relationship: challenges and recommendations. *International Review of Psychiatry*, **23: 10–19.**

Rorty, R. (1987) Science as solidarity. In *The Rhetoric of the Human Sciences: Language and Argument in Scholarship and Public Affairs* (eds J. S. Nelson, A. Megill & D. N. McCloskey), pp. 38–52. University of Wisconsin Press.

Rose, N. (1998) *Inventing our Selves: Psychology, Power, and Personhood*. Cambridge University Press.

Sadavoy, J., Meier, R., Amoy Yuk Mui Ong, R. (2004) Barriers to access to mental health services for ethnic seniors: the Toronto Study. *Canadian Journal of Psychiatry*, **49**, 192–199.

Shobe, M. A., Coffman, M. J. & Dmochowski, J. (2009) Achieving the American dream: facilitators and barriers to health and mental health for Latino immigrants. *Journal of Evidence-Based Social Work*, **6**, 92–110.

Singh, N. N., McKay, J. D. & Singh, A. N. (1998) Culture and mental health: nonverbal communication. *Journal of Child and Family Studies*, **7**, 403–409.

Skelton, J. R., Kai, J. & Loudon, R. F. (2001) Cross-cultural communication in medicine: questions for educators. *Medical Education*, **35**, 257–261.

Sue, S. (2003) In defense of cultural competency in psychotherapy and treatment. *American Psychologist*, **58**, 964–970.

Sue, D. W. & Sue, D. (1977) Barriers to effective cross-cultural counseling. *Journal of Counseling Psychology*, **24**, 420–429.

Sue, D. W. & Sue, D. (1999) *Counseling the Culturally Different: Theory and Practice* (3rd edn). John Wiley & Sons.

Ulrey, K. L. & Amason, P. (2001) Intercultural communication between patients and health care providers: exploration of intercultural communication effectiveness, cultural sensitivity, stress, and anxiety. *Health Communication*, **13**, 449–463.

Van Wieringen, J. C. M., Harmsen, J. Á. M. & Brujnzeels, M. A. (2002) Intercultural communication in general practice. *European Journal of Public Health*, **12**, 63–68.

Walls, G. B. (2004) Toward a critical global psychoanalysis. *Psychoanalytic Dialogues: The International Journal of Relational Perspectives*, **14**, 605–634.

Watkins, C. E., Terrell, F., Miller, F. S., *et al* (1989) Cultural mistrust and its effects on expectational variables in Black client–White counselor relationships. *Journal of Counseling Psychology*, **36**, 447–450.

Welch, I. D. (2003) *The Therapeutic Relationship: Listening and Responding in a Multicultural World*. Praeger Publishers.

Whaley, A. L. (1998) Racism in the provision of mental health services: a social-cognitive analysis. *American Journal of Orthopsychiatry*, **68**, 47–57.

Whaley, A. L. (2001) Cultural mistrust and mental health services for African Americans. *Counseling Psychologist*, **29**, 513–531.

Wrenn, C. G. (1985) Afterword: the culturally encapsulated counselor revisited. In *Handbook of Cross-Cultural Counseling and Therapy* (ed. P. B. Pedersen), pp. 323–330. Greenwood Press.

Wu, M. C., Kviz, F. J. & Miller, A. M. (2009) Identifying individual and contextual barriers to seeking mental health services among Korean American immigrant women. *Issues in Mental Health Nursing*, **30**, 78–85.

Yi, K. (1995) Psychoanalytic psychotherapy with Asian clients: transference and therapeutic consideration. *Psychotherapy*, **32**, 308–314.

CHAPTER 12

How does intercultural interpretation work in the mental health setting?

Rachel Tribe and Adil Qureshi

Please ask yourself the following questions, then return to them after you have read this chapter, to see whether you wish to reconsider any of your responses:

- What exactly is intercultural interpretation in the mental health setting?
- What is expected of the interpreter?
- What is being interpreted or mediated in such an encounter?
- Each individual brings their own culture into a meeting, which is itself mediated by a number of factors at the micro- (individual) and macro- (cultural and contextual) level. Is it merely language that is being interpreted or is it something more complex, which includes culture, world views and explanatory health beliefs?
- Is it possible to work effectively with an interpreter to ensure that a patient's mental health needs are addressed appropriately and respectfully?

The challenges

There can be resistance to, or difficulties associated with, working through an interpreter, including feelings of threat and possible exposure experienced by all parties (Westermeyer, 1990). The overall and transferential dynamics within the meeting may be changed (Tribe & Thompson, 2009; Qureshi *et al*, 2011). Psychiatrists may feel a lack of experience in working through interpreters and may have concerns about how it will affect the meeting and about the accuracy of the interpreting. Patients may be very worried that their words and emotions may not be communicated adequately (Tribe & Raval, 2003). The interpreter may have concerns about working within a psychiatric setting (Razban, 2003). Lack of training and support for interpreters is a matter of concern. They may not be trained in mental health, nor be receiving support or clinical supervision, leaving them vulnerable to vicarious traumatisation (Doherty *et al*, 2010). We must not assume that a patient and interpreter who share a language will also share a culture. The latter is highly individualistic and there can be dangers in assuming any commonality of culture between interpreter and client. Language and culture interact in complex ways, and the interpreter may be negotiating between three world views: the patient's, the clinician's and their own (Drennan & Swartz, 1999).

Solutions

There are many advantages to working through an interpreter and it is a skill that should be in the repertoire of all psychiatrists. Training for interpreters on working in mental health and for psychiatrists on working in collaboration with interpreters is needed to improve the experience for all members of the triad and to ensure good outcomes from the consultation. The presence of an interpreter can actively enhance matters by enabling the psychiatrist to do their job, encouraging reflection, the consideration of other cultural perspectives, explanatory health beliefs, idioms of distress and cultural taboos, and a questioning of assumptions that may be culturally located (Raval, 1996). It can also appropriately normalise the experience of a mental health encounter for the patient (Pezous, 1992) and show that diversity is considered within the service.

Working effectively with an interpreter ensures that people who are not fluent in English can access psychiatric services and good-quality care based on a thorough assessment. Protecting the principles of equality backed up by legislation (such as the UK's Equality Act 2010) should ensure this. This is in line with Department of Health directives. Many of the advantages of working through an interpreter have been noted by Farooq & Fear (2003). The presence of an interpreter or intercultural mediator can lead to better clinical outcomes (Eytan *et al*, 2002), and experienced interpreters provide reliable data for diagnosis by the clinician (Farooq *et al*, 1997). Interpreters can themselves act as cultural mediators (Qureshi *et al*, 2011). A systematic review of the literature on the use of interpreters for patients with limited English proficiency revealed that professional interpreters were associated with greater improvements in clinical care than were *ad hoc* interpreters, and that professional interpreters were able to raise care to a level comparable to that received by language-proficient patients (Karliner *et al*, 2007).

Recommendations for practice

- Undertake a language needs analysis for your local population and consider how you will best meet this need.
- Undertake training. A possible training curriculum can be found in Tribe & Raval (2003). If you have to work through an interpreter unexpectedly, discuss this with a more experienced colleague.

- Check that the interpreter is qualified and appropriate for the consultation.
- If there is more than one meeting, ensure that the same interpreter is used throughout.
- Allocate 10–15 minutes in advance of the session to brief the interpreter about the purpose of the meeting and to enable them to brief you about any cultural issues that may have bearing on the session. At the end of the session, debrief the interpreter about the session and offer support and supervision as appropriate.
- Be curious about and interested in other constructions of the issues people bring.
- Be mindful of issues of confidentiality and trust when working with someone from a small language community.
- State clearly that you alone hold clinical responsibility for the meeting.
- Create a congenial atmosphere where each member of the triad feels able to ask for clarification.
- Be respectful to your interpreter.
- Match when appropriate for gender and age, do not use a relative and never use a child.
- Consider the well-being of your interpreter and the potential for vicarious traumatisation; consider what support will be offered.
- All translated written material used should have been back-translated.
- Caution should be exercised when considering the use of translated psychometric tests.
- Commissioners need to ensure that there are clear pathways to support for all members of their local community, including those who do not speak English.

References and further reading

Antinucci, G. (2004) Another language, another place: to hide or be found. *International Journal of Psychoanalysis*, **85**, 1157–1173.

British Psychological Society (2008) Working with Interpreters in Health Settings: Guidelines for Psychologists. BPS Professional Affairs Board (http://www.bps.org.uk/content/working-interpreters-health-settings).

Department of Health & University of East London (2011) *Interpretation in Mental Health Settings: A Quick Guide* (DVD). Department of Health & University of East London (http://www.youtube.com/watch?v=k0wzhakyjck).

Doherty, S., MacIntyre A. M. & Wyne, T. (2010) How does it feel for you? The emotional impact and specific challenges of mental health interpreting. *Mental Health Review Journal*, **15**, 31–44.

Drennan, G. & Swartz, L. (1999) A concept overburdened: institutional roles for psychiatric interpreters in post-apartheid South Africa. *Interpreting*, **4**, 169–198.

Eytan, A., Bischoff, A., Rrustemi, I., *et al* (2002) Screening of mental disorders in asylum-seekers from Kosovo. *Australian and New Zealand Journal of Psychiatry*, **36**, 499–503.

Farooq, S. & Fear, C. (2003) Working through interpreters. *Advances in Psychiatric Treatment*, **9**, 104–109.

Farooq, S., Fear, C. F. & Oyebode, F. (1997) An investigation of the adequacy of psychiatric interviews conducted through an interpreter. *Psychiatric Bulletin*, **21**, 209–213.

Karliner, L. S., Jacobs, E. A., Chen, A. H., *et al* (2007) Do professional interpreters improve clinical care for patients with limited English proficiency? A systematic review of the literature. *Health Services Research*, **42**, 727–754.

Lewis, M. P. (ed.) (2009) *Ethnologue: Languages of the World* (16th edn). SIL International. (http://www.ethnologue.com).

Pezous, A. (1992) A propos d'une experience clinique psychiatrique dans un camp de réfugiés Khmers en Thailande. *Annales Psychiatriques*, **7**, 151–155.

Qureshi, A., Revollo, H-W., Collazos, F., *et al* (2011) Intercultural mediation: reconstructing Hermes – the messenger gets a voice. In *Migration and Mental Health* (eds D. Bhugra & S. Gupta), pp. 245–260. Cambridge University Press.

Raval, H. (1996) A systemic perspective on working with interpreters. *Clinical Child Psychology and Psychiatry*, **1**, 29–43.

Razban, M. (2003) An interpreter's perspective. In *Undertaking Mental Health Work Using Interpreters* (eds R. Tribe & H. Raval), pp. 92–98. Brunner-Routledge.

Tribe, R. & Raval, H. (eds) (2003) *Working with Interpreters in Mental Health*. Brunner-Routledge.

Tribe, R. & Thompson, K. (2009) Exploring the three-way relationship in therapeutic work with interpreters. *International Journal of Migration, Health and Social Care*, **5**, 13–21.

Westermeyer, J. (1990) Working with an interpreter in psychiatric assessment and treatment. *Journal of Nervous and Mental Disease*, **178**, 745–749.

CHAPTER 13

Do the power relations inherent in medical systems help or hinder in cross-cultural psychiatry?

Peter Ferns, Premila Trivedi and Suman Fernando

Power relations are a structural characteristic of all social relationships, organisational systems and societies as a whole (Proctor, 2002; Dalal, 2003). Certain identities are accorded different powers and status depending on who they are as people (societal, personal and historic power) and the position they hold within a hierarchical institution or work setting (role-power; authority). In medicine, doctors (because of their education, training, experience and expertise) have the authority to diagnose and treat those they deem to be ill, with clear boundaries, systems of accountability and opportunities for others to challenge those decisions if there are breaches of a doctor's defined roles. Less obvious perhaps is the societal, personal and historic powers exerted (often unwittingly) by doctors' values, biases and assumptions about their patients, since subjectivity is part of the clinical task. These informal values and systemic biases are not easy to identify, not necessarily limited by any formal boundaries and have no regulated system of accountability, leaving their influence to the discretion of each individual clinician. This source of influence and power is of particular significance in psychiatry, where diagnosis and treatment are determined not by an objective measurement or scientific test or biomarker, but rather by professional judgements that make positive and creative use of subjectivity (Loring & Powell, 1988; Fernando, 2010).

Psychiatry is firmly located within medical systems of authority, developed (at least initially) within Western (Euro–American, industrialised and high-income) countries and cultures; within these cultures, doctors were allocated the authority to name problematic thoughts, feelings and behaviours as illness of the mind (see Chapter 14, this volume). However, aspects of these problematic thoughts, feelings and behaviours are culturally determined and they may fall outside psychiatry's Eurocentric frame of reference. They may, however, be acceptable within their relevant cultural contexts. In such situations, misunderstandings can easily occur when psychiatrists (wittingly or unwittingly) use not only authority but also power in a way that is at least partially determined by their personal values and biases to inform diagnosis, risk assessment, treatment and management (Loring & Powell, 1988). The effects of this can be very serious and reach far beyond the confines of medicine, since psychiatrists have the authority to use medical, social, psychological, behavioural and physical interventions (by coercion if they deem this necessary). At the most worrying end of this spectrum of activity there may be grave breaches of patients' human and civil rights (Inyama, 2009). Ways of limiting the adverse effects of psychiatric power and authority relations and of enabling these to be applied in fairer and more positive ways form an important part of psychiatry in practice. Yet direct discussion of power and authority relations is often sidelined in psychiatric discourse (Tew, 2005). Instead, the focus is on differences in race and culture to account for the way certain racialised groups are diagnosed and treated within psychiatry and on psychiatry's beneficent medical intentions rather than the very real consequences of its actions. A silence is thus created that not only normalises the ways in which power and authority are used in psychiatry, but also restricts opportunities to explore how these could be used in much more positive ways to open up possibilities for change and achievement (Foucault 1980, 1984).

Ways forward

From the above discussion it may appear that power and authority in psychiatry are largely in the possession of psychiatrists, unidirectional and static. However, using post-structural concepts, Proctor (2002) has described power and authority as being not in the possession of one person but rather in the relationship, bidirectional and dynamic. Evidence of this can clearly be seen in the experiences of psychiatric patients who, while they may lack authority in psychiatric settings, certainly have power. In an excellent chapter on power relations in mental healthcare, Tew (2005: p. 72) has stated that 'in seemingly powerless situations, people may develop strategies for survival and become adept at resisting or subverting the expectations that may be made of them, or the identities that may be placed on them, often in subtle and even unconscious ways. Such manoeuvres, sometimes seen as being "difficult" or "manipulative" by those in positions of relative dominance, may nevertheless represent service users' most realistic strategies for having any influence on their situation'.

Knowing that things cannot get any worse can (at times) be marvellously freeing and, as a service user explains, using their physical power to kick in the ward office door can generate an immediate flash of empowerment – until they are once more plunged into the depths of subjugation and disempowerment by being controlled and restrained with no attempt to find out the reasons for their actions (Trivedi, 2002).

But this sets up a dynamic which is risk-laden for all. For psychiatrists, using their authority to diagnose illness (which has no biochemical or other physical markers), manage human distress (which all too frequently arises as a result of socioeconomic rather than medical 'factors'), carry out risk assessments (which can never be 100% accurate) and enable both psychiatric patients and the public to feel safe (which is often impossible to achieve simultaneously) will inevitably result in feelings of stress, frustration and defensiveness. For patients, using their power in an attempt to overcome feelings of invalidation and disempowerment, a sense of hopelessness and fear of legally sanctioned violence and then being further disempowered will also result in stress and defensiveness. This creates a situation in which both parties get caught up in a vicious circle of trying to assert power over one another, with mutual attempts at domination and lack of meaningful communication or relationship (O'Brien & O'Brien, 1994).

One way to overcome this may be for psychiatrists to use their power and authority in more positive ways; for example, in 'power-with' mode rather than 'power-over' mode. Power-with mode is much more about dignity and respect, meaningful communication and positive relationship, partnership working with mutual learning and negotiation (O'Brien & O'Brien, 1994). But this is not as easy as it sounds, particularly in cross-cultural settings. Here, psychiatrists must have the ability and willingness to use their power and authority to: (a) look at problems through the eyes of the people who use services, especially if they come from cultural backgrounds that are unfamiliar to the psychiatrists; and (b) make allowances for their own prejudices and the limitations of judgements – and hence diagnoses – that are made in cross-cultural encounters. Using authority and power in this power-with mode will be more challenging and time-consuming for psychiatrists, but for service users it will be massively beneficial and lead to much better outcomes. Most important, being aware of power relations and consciously attempting to use power positively will be a reminder that:

- there is nothing wrong with power and authority in themselves: it is how they are used that is important
- power and authority can be used to either oppress or liberate
- there is always a choice.

Conclusion

We conclude that neither the power derived from naming 'illness' nor the authority vested in mental health professionals to judge the risk of social danger in instances where diagnoses are made are likely to disappear in the foreseeable future. If psychiatrists wish to work ethically within the system, it behoves them to recognise as an inherent part of their work that power and authority must be used positively with patients and to make every effort to work round the often discriminatory systems they are placed in, so that they interfere as little as possible in the lives of their patients.

References

Dalal, F. (2003) Power: the generator of difference. In *Race, Colour and the Process of Racialization: New Perspectives from Group Analysis, Psychoanalysis and Sociology* (ed. F. Dalal), pp. 120–134. Brunner-Routledge.

Fernando, S. (2010) *Mental Health, Race and Culture*. Palgrave-Macmillan.

Foucault, M. (1980) *Power/Knowledge: Selected Interviews and Other Writings 1972–1977* (ed. C. Gordon). Pantheon Books.

Foucault, M. (1984) Space, knowledge, and power: an interview with Michel Foucault conducted by Paul Rabinow. In *The Foucault Reader* (ed. P. Rabinow), pp. 239–256. Penguin Books.

Inyama, C. (2009) Race relations, mental health and human rights – the legal framework. In *Mental Health in a Multi-Ethnic Society: A Multidisciplinary Handbook* (2nd edn) (eds S. Fernando & F. Keating), pp. 27–41. Routledge.

Loring, M. & Powell, B. (1988) Gender, race and DSM-III: a study of the objectivity of psychiatric diagnostic behavior. *Journal of Health and Social Behavior*, **29**, 1–22.

O'Brien, J. & O'Brien, C. L. (1994) *More Than Just a New Address: Images of Organization for Supported Living Agencies*. Responsive Systems Associates (http://www.mnddc.org/parallels2/pdf/90s/91/91-MTA-RSA.pdf).

Proctor G. (2002) *The Dynamics of Power in Counselling and Psychotherapy: Ethics, Politics and Practice*. PCCS Books.

Tew, J. (2005) Power relations, social order and mental distress. In *Social Perspectives in Mental Health: Developing Social Models to Understand and Work with Mental Distress* (ed. J. Tew), pp. 71–89. Jessica Kingsley.

Trivedi, P. (2002) Racism, social exclusion and mental health. In *Racism and Mental Health*. (ed. K. Bhui), pp. 71–82. Jessica Kingsley.

CHAPTER 14

Recovery and well-being: a paradigm for care

Suman Fernando, Premila Trivedi and Peter Ferns

The World Health Organization (2001: p. 3) defines health as 'a state of complete physical, mental and social well-being'. What is meant to any individual by well-being, mental health and what constitute mental health problems, and to some extent mental illness, is largely determined by the cultural and social circumstances of communities in which the individual in most instances is immersed (Fernando, 2010). In multicultural situations, different interpretations exist side by side, but which ones dominate will be determined by the power relations that exist between the different cultural groups (see Chapter 13, this volume). The closest we can get to studying well-being and mental health as experienced by people in particular cultural/multicultural and social settings is therefore to explore not only the meanings that are given by each constituent community, but also how some meanings are privileged over others and how this can serve to diminish or invalidate others. By the same argument, the meaning of recovery from mental health problems must also be defined within specific cultural/multicultural and social contexts.

The terms well-being and mental health capture different concepts: the former encompasses personal, social and spiritual aspects of life and functioning in society, whereas the latter implies a biomedical understanding of how a person's mind functions. The focus on well-being has grown rapidly in recent years and is justified on the grounds that, in contrast to assessments of mental health by experts, well-being: (a) is based on standards and values chosen by people themselves; (b) reflects success or failure in achieving norms and values that people themselves seek; and (c) includes components dependent on pleasure and the fulfilment of basic human needs, but also includes people's ethical and evaluative judgements of their lives (Diener & Suh, 2000). At a personal level, well-being, sometimes called subjective well-being or happiness (Diener, 1984), is a positive state of mind brought about by satisfaction of personal, relational and collective needs (Prilleltensky et al, 2001). However, there is another approach (the capabilities approach) to well-being, which is more about what people can *do* as agents and *are* in terms of lived experience – the emphasis being on their having the capability (i.e. the practical choice) to function (Sen, 2008). We suggest that well-being in a broad sense is more meaningful as a concept than the narrow term mental health, which is seemingly located in one part, one aspect, of the human being.

Like well-being, recovery has also grown in importance in psychiatry in recent years (Care Services Improvement Partnership *et al*, 2007) as an alternative to the narrow symptom-based approach to clinical practice, and it now underpins most mental health policy documents. However, it is crucial to remember where the concept of recovery originated: service users (often battling against the authority of psychiatry) introduced the concept in mental health to describe personal journeys in which they follow their personally (not professionally) defined goals, making sense of their experiences, gaining a greater understanding of themselves and their environments, taking power into their own hands and, above all, creating hope for a better future (Sayce & Perkins, 2000; Repper & Perkins, 2003). This individual-centred recovery concept has developed in the West and therefore has limitations for people from a non-Western cultural background, especially those facing discrimination and social exclusion (Social Perspectives Network, 2007). Over time, concepts of recovery developed by service users have been taken up/taken over by mental health systems (providers, professionals and policy makers) and a recovery approach moulded to fit in with their already established structures and norms (Trivedi, 2010). Such an approach is in danger of becoming as negative as previous approaches, with many service users equating a recovery approach with loss of services, loss of benefits and a push towards returning to work, without the support, retraining and flexibility this would require (Wallcraft, 2010). For service users from Black and minority ethnic (BME) communities, there are also particular issues in applying an approach based on Western concepts of recovery; for them, a recovery journey will be not only about recovery from mental health experiences, but also about circumventing or overcoming barriers of a social and political nature which have contributed to their mental health problems in the first place. Such a journey will involve connecting with family, religion and community, and possibly political movements. In such situations, the term recovery may be too mild and the journey needs to be better represented by a word such as liberation.

These issues concerning the concept of recovery and how it is being implemented should be seen in the context of a subtle power struggle regarding recovery that is emerging in the British mental health scene between, on the one hand, professional systemic power of the medical establishment and, on the other, the voice of service users and like-minded people (Fernando, 2010). This struggle is not necessary. Concepts of well-being and recovery together could form an alternative to the diagnosis–assessment–treatment approach of traditional biomedical psychiatry, and be much better suited to the needs of a multicultural society. Thus, in clinical practice in British multicultural settings, it may be preferable for psychiatrists to limit their use of traditional psychiatry and use instead in most circumstances a recovery–well-being–liberation focused model. People focusing on racism and cultural issues in delivery of services appear as a third dimension in this struggle, but it is often difficult to determine where exactly they are placed since they (especially BME service users) seem to be largely absent from official debates on recovery (Trivedi, 2008; Fernando, 2010). However, if a more inclusive debate can begin, if power relations can be honestly considered and the concept of recovery allowed to develop in a more authentic and holistic way, it may offer a shift in the culture of psychiatry that would be much more hopeful for the people it serves.

Some critical questions

- Who defines recovery and controls the recovery process in your service – the professionals or the service users and their carers?
- Are the approaches taken to diagnosis, assessment and treatment sufficiently flexible to be applied across cultures?
- Are recovery approaches in your services systemic as well as individualised, i.e. do they consider family and community needs as well as individual needs?

References and further reading

Care Services Improvement Partnership, Royal College of Psychiatrists & Social Care Institute for Excellence (2007) *A Common Purpose: Recovery in Future Mental Health Services* (Joint Position Paper 08). SCIE (http://www.scie.org.uk/publications/positionpapers/pp08.pdf).

Davidson, L., Rakfeldt, J. & Strauss, J. (eds) (2010) *The Roots of the Recovery Movement in Psychiatry: Lessons Learned*. Wiley-Blackwell.

Department of Health (2009) *New Horizons: Towards a Shared Vision for Mental Health*. Department of Health.

Diener, E. (1984) Subjective well-being. *Psychological Bulletin*, **96**, 542–575.

Diener, E. & Suh, E. M. (2000) Measuring subjective well-being to compare quality of life of cultures. In *Culture and Subjective Well-being* (eds E. Diener & E. M. Suh), pp. 3–12. MIT Press.

Fernando, S. (2010) *Mental Health, Race and Culture* (3rd edn). Palgrave Macmillan.

Prilleltensky, I., Nelson, G. & Peirson, L. (2001) *Promoting Family Wellness and Preventing Child Maltreatment: Fundamentals for Thinking and Action*. University of Toronto Press.

Repper, J. & Perkins, R. (2003) *Social Inclusion and Recovery: A Model for Mental Health Practice*. Ballière Tindall.

Sayce, E. & Perkins, R. (2000) Recovery: beyond mere survival. *Psychiatric Bulletin*, **24**, 74–75.

Sen, A. (2008) Economics of happiness and capability. In *Capabilities and Happiness* (eds L. Bruni, F. Comim & M. Pugno), pp. 16–27. Oxford University Press.

Social Perspectives Network (2007) *Whose Recovery is it Anyway?* (SPN Paper 11). SPN.

Trivedi, P. (2008) Black service 'user involvement' – rhetoric or reality? In *Mental Health in a Multi-Ethnic Society: A Multidisciplinary Handbook* (eds S. Fernando & F. Keating), pp. 136–146. Routledge.

Trivedi, P. (2010) A recovery approach in mental health services: transformation, tokenism or tyranny? In *Voices of Experience* (eds T. Bassett & T. Stickley), pp. 152–163. Wiley-Blackwell.

Wallcraft, J. (2010) The Capabilities Approach in mental health: what are the implications for research and outcome measurement? Presentation to the General Assembly of the European Network of Users and Survivors in Psychiatry, Thessaloniki, 30 September 2010 (http://www.slideserve.com/libitha/the-capabilities-approach-in-mental-health).

World Health Organization (2001) *The World Health Report 2001. Mental Health: New Understanding, New Hope*. WHO (http://www.who.int/whr/2001/en/whr01_en.pdf).

CHAPTER 15

Social perspectives on diagnosis

Premila Trivedi, Suman Fernando and Peter Ferns

Modern Western psychology and psychiatry arose in the context of the European Enlightenment of the 17th and 18th centuries. In the early 19th century, only two main mental illnesses were usually recognised – mania and melancholia (Shorter, 1997). As various theories of mental functioning came on the scene, new diagnoses were constructed in Europe and North America and two key diagnostic systems, the International Classification of Diseases (ICD) and Diagnostic and Statistical Manual of Mental Disorders (DSM), were developed. These are revised from time to time by groups of psychiatrists mainly living in the West and usually strongly influenced by pressure groups, including pharmaceutical companies wishing to market new remedies for illnesses. The first DSM (American Psychiatric Association, 1952) contained 60 diagnoses; the current edition, DSM-IV (American Psychiatric Association, 1994), lists 297; and DSM-5, to be published in 2013, is likely to have even more (American Psychiatric Association, 2010).

A few diagnoses have fallen by the wayside. For example, gone are several popularised in the southern states of the USA as peculiar to Black slaves, such as drapetomania, characterised by persistent running away from the plantations (Cartwright, 1851). Homosexuality was listed as an illness in the DSM until the seventh printing of DSM-IV in 1974 and in the ICD until ICD-10, published in 1990 (Shorter, 1997). Well into the 1960s, depression was reported as rare among Asian and African people and Black Americans, a rarity attributed to their supposed irresponsible nature (Green, 1914) and absence of a sense of responsibility (Carothers, 1953).

A multi-ethnic society includes people whose backgrounds are culturally diverse as well as people seen as different in terms of race. No psychiatric diagnosis has an established biological marker; hence, there is no way of proving objectively its accuracy or its validity as a measure of a biological reality applicable to all human beings. Kendell & Jablensky (2003) describe diagnostic categories as 'simply concepts, justified only by whether they provide a useful framework for organizing and explaining the complexity of clinical experience in order to derive inferences about outcome and to guide decisions about treatment'. They warn against reifying a diagnosis by assuming that it is 'an entity of some kind that can be evoked to explain the patient's symptoms and whose validity need not be questioned'. The basic problem inherent in using Western psychiatric diagnoses across cultures may be conceptualised as category fallacy – the error of using a diagnostic category derived in one cultural context to identify illness in another culture (Kleinman, 1977). However, the problems in clinical practice and research are much wider than just diagnostic issues. Cultural diversity in people's world views and variation in the meanings they give to health and illness, and to the mind itself, are all reflected in cross-cultural clinical work (see the vast literature referred to in, for example, Fernando, 2010). So, to ensure greater accuracy in the diagnostic process, it is essential to establish a wider basis for diagnosis, that incorporates cultural and social perspectives.

Apart from culture, another issue that plays into diagnostic anomalies is 'race thinking', described by Barzun (1965, p. x) as 'singling out certain traits that are observed, accurately or not, in one or more individuals, and making of these traits a composite character which is then assumed to be uniform, or at least prevailing throughout the group'. One of the few well-conducted studies into racial and gender bias in the diagnostic habits of psychiatrists was reported by Loring & Powell (1988) in the USA. They used carefully selected case studies, manipulating them so that approximately one-fifth of the clinicians evaluated a White male, one-fifth a White female, one-fifth a Black male, one-fifth a Black female, and one-fifth a client whose gender and

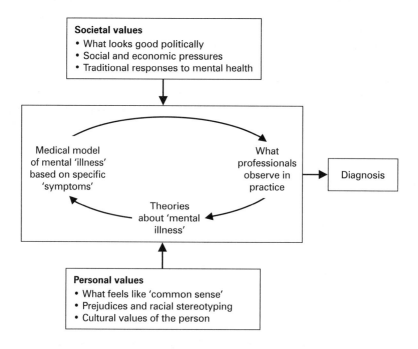

Fig. 15.1 The societal context of diagnosis (© 2010, Peter Ferns).

race were not disclosed. The researchers found that: (a) overall, compared with White clients, Black clients were given a diagnosis of schizophrenia more frequently by both Black and White clinicians – although to a lesser extent by the former; and (b) in their additional comments on the case studies, all the clinicians appeared to ascribe violence, suspiciousness and dangerousness to Black clients, even though the case studies were the same as those for the White clients. Loring & Powell concluded that Black and White people are 'seen differentially even if they exhibit the same behaviour and that these differences are reflected and legitimized in official statistics on psychopathology'. This is a demonstration of the power exerted by the personal values and biases of professionals in shaping diagnosis.

The main problem in clinical work is that stereotypes about Black people – for instance, regarding violence, anger and dangerousness – pervade images and ideas prevalent in society, feeding into the judgements that go to make up the diagnostic process. The efforts of psychiatrists and others in mental healthcare to be culturally sensitive and anti-racist may attenuate these effects but are unlikely to obviate them. Most research is medically driven. It therefore tends to avoid investigating institutional practices (including the diagnostic process), focusing instead on head counts of people already diagnosed or on examining the opinions and judgements of professionals, while accepting diagnoses themselves as valid indicators of mental health problems.

In multicultural settings or in situations in which psychiatric diagnoses are applied across cultures, it is essential that the limitations of diagnosis are borne in mind at all stages of psychiatric practice. In many instances, it may be necessary to ignore diagnosis altogether and to assess patients from a social perspective alone, focusing on their narratives rather than relying on traditions of gathering a psychiatric history that may overlook the patient's perspective. Moreover, service users' needs, interests and hopes for the future may become the primary focus for practice, with psychiatric intervention contributing through a recovery-based approach (see Chapter 14, this volume).

Some critical questions

- Why is a social model approach to diagnosis more useful in dealing with patients who are vulnerable to institutional discrimination?
- What impact would a social model approach to diagnosis have on the power dynamics that usually operate between clinicians, patients and their families?

References and further reading

American Psychiatric Association (1952) *Diagnostic and Statistical Manual of Mental Disorders*. APA.

American Psychiatric Association (1994) *Diagnostic and Statistical Manual of Mental Disorders (4th edn) (DSM–IV)*. APA.

American Psychiatric Association (2010) *Proposed Draft Revisions to DSM Disorders and Criteria*. APA (http://www.dsm5.org/ProposedRevisions/Pages/Default.aspx).

Barzun, J. (1965) *Race: A Study in Superstition*. Harper & Row.

Carothers, J. C. (1953) *The African Mind in Health and Disease: A Study in Ethnopsychiatry*. World Health Organization.

Cartwright, S. A. (1851) Report on the diseases and physical peculiarities of the Negro race. Reprinted (1981) in Concepts of Health and Disease (eds A. C. Caplan, H. T. Engelhardt and J. J. McCartney), pp. 305–325. Addison-Wesley.

Fernando, S. (2010) *Mental Health, Race and Culture* (3rd edn). Palgrave Macmillan.

Gaines, A. D. (ed.) *Ethnopsychiatry: The Cultural Construction of Professional and Folk Psychiatries*. State University of New York Press.

Green, E. M. (1914) Psychoses among Negroes – a comparative study. *Journal of Nervous and Mental Disorder*, **41**, 697–708.

Kendell, R. & Jablensky, A. (2003) Distinguishing between the validity and utility of psychiatric diagnoses. *American Journal of Psychiatry*, **160**, 4–12.

Kleinman, A. (1977) Depression, somatization and the 'new cross-cultural psychiatry'. *Social Science and Medicine*, **11**, 3–10.

Kuhn, T. S. (1996) *The Structure of Scientific Revolutions* (3rd edn). University of Chicago Press.

Loring, M. & Powell, B. (1988) Gender, race and DSM-III: a study of the objectivity of psychiatric diagnostic behavior. *Journal of Health and Social Behavior*, **29**, 1–22.

Marsella, A. J. & White, G. M. (eds) (1984) *Cultural Conceptions of Mental Health and Therapy*. Reidel.

Obeyesekere, G. (1985) Depression, Buddhism, and the work of culture in Sri Lanka. In *Culture and Depression: Studies in the Anthropology and Cross-Cultural Psychiatry of Affect and Disorder* (eds A. Kleinman & B. Good), pp. 134–152. University of California Press.

Shorter, E. (1997) *A History of Psychiatry: From the Era of Asylum to the Age of Prozac*. John Wiley & Sons.

CHAPTER 16

Public mental health and inequalities

Kamaldeep Bhui

A strong case for a public mental health strategy exists, given the benefits to society as a whole and to those with mental health problems. This approach requires universal interventions applied to the entire population, such that the benefits are available to the greatest number of people (Rose, 1992). The idea is to not restrict interventions only to people who have developed an illness, leaving health risks in the rest of the population unaddressed. An example of the strategy is the recent emphasis on well-being and happiness, and on symptoms of anxiety, depression and psychosis in the population that do not meet diagnostic criteria but are associated with disabilities (e.g. van Os *et al*, 2009; Rai *et al*, 2010). Effective interventions that can be used in preventive psychiatry or public mental health include preventing violence and abuse in early life and preventing age- and gender-based violence and discrimination throughout the lifespan. This would create a more balanced and empowering society in which all adults, regardless of their age, gender and cultural background, could realise their potential in the workplace and avoid long periods of sickness and illness-related absence from work. Information should be available for the population on how to maximise their good health and prevent illness by taking lifestyle, behavioural, social, psychological and physical measures. It should include not only how to minimise the impact of illness, but also how to prevent it arising, especially for groups who appear to be at high risk. Many of these interventions aim to act over the life course, protecting and promoting what has been called mental capital (Jenkins *et al*, 2008).

To some extent mental health professionals, including psychiatrists, are already undertaking activities that have a preventive function (Box 16.1).

Inequalities

The public health approach does not explicitly address ethnic or cultural inequalities of service use and experience. However, the aim of public health policy is to avoid the development of inequalities in general by ensuring that illness is prevented in the first place, specifically by tackling the social determinants of illness, which are unequally patterned. The

---

Box 16.1   Examples of public mental health activities

- Prevention to protect mental health, either by delaying onset or minimising disability, illness episodes, loss of social networks and financial strain
- Providing models and methods to work with hard-to-reach groups, in order they benefit from public health interventions; this will require some targeting
- Providing models and methods to work with risk behaviours and prevention: violence, self-harm, eating disorders, depression, anxiety, workplace stress, relational issues
- Preventing poor health amongst those with mental health problems by encouraging take up of public health messages and interventions and specifically to minimise the health burden (beyond mental health) encountered
- Preventing extreme life events with long-term mental health burden: violence, abuse
- Promoting positive mental health strategies over the life course: for children – learning, risk behaviours, friendships, coping with loss, understanding parental illness; for the elderly – working with memory and sustaining employment; for all – exercise and physical activity, nutrition, well-being and happiness, self-esteem and confidence, self-efficacy

---

public health approach can remove inequalities by addressing social and material circumstances, education and employment opportunities. Other approaches in policy and legislation address stigma and discrimination in the workplace and in society in general.

The risk of such an approach is that some in society are less able to hear about related initiatives, to take them up or to adhere to them. These include individuals with poorer educational and social status, those who find it hard to change a lifestyle that already compromises their health, those who already have severe health problems and those who are socially excluded and have multiple problems. The last group includes homeless populations, those exposed to discrimination or stigma and, of course, people with severe mental illness. All of these groups may consequently fall even further behind in terms of health improvements, so that the inequality gap widens rather than narrows, albeit that absolute levels of illness may not decline, unless the new programmes divert resources away from high-risk and socially excluded groups.

This issue is not confined to people with mental health problems. It has also been raised in other areas of medicine, for example, cardiovascular medicine (Capewell & Graham, 2010). Therefore, targeted interventions are necessary for those who are less likely to benefit from a universal approach. It is possible that the emphasis on young people in such endeavours may inadvertently discriminate against older populations, so actions are needed to embrace preventive approaches among the latter. The absence of mention in public health policy of discrimination on the basis of race, ethnicity, religion and culture in part reflects the broad ambition of policy to be overarching. However, this absence of focus on specific groups risks failing those whose health concerns are perhaps already being overlooked and will be neglected to a greater extent. Such oversight is common to offender patients, people with intellectual disability, older people, refugees and asylum seekers, homeless populations, and lesbian, gay, bisexual and transgendered people. Each of these groups will require specific consideration and roll out of policies and actions for engagement that improve their health status and prevent illness. When equality is discussed, it tends to raise concerns about resources, about social justice and about how to tackle such matters. These concerns can fuel disagreement about the relevance of race and ethnicity and calls for more evidence, while halting or reversing previous agreement and actions to tackle these issues. Such regressive actions can be seen relatively easily when change is expected of providers, commissioners and policy makers (Wilson, 2009; Bhui *et al*, 2012). Public mental health actions at population level should not undermine or remove action at service, commissioner and individual practitioner levels. There are still substantial inequalities in mental healthcare and this should remain a priority. The challenge for commissioners, providers and practitioners is to not destroy the good work that has gone on for many decades in improving practitioners' knowledge, skills and attitudes and in bolstering the evidence base for healthcare provision to diverse cultural groups (Wilson, 2009). Many of the mechanisms of therapeutic failure or treatment breakdown that are discussed in other chapters in this book can be discerned at organisational and societal levels.

References

Bhui, K., Ascoli, M. & Nuamh, O. (2012) The place of race and racism in cultural competence: what can we learn from the English experience about the narratives of evidence and argument? *Transcultural Psychiatry*, **49**, 185–205.

Capewell, S. & Graham, H. (2010) Will cardiovascular disease prevention widen health inequalities? *Plos Medicine*, **7**(8), e1000320.

Jenkins, R., Meltzer, H., Jones, P. B., *et al* (2008) *Foresight Mental Capital and Wellbeing Project. Mental Health: Future Challenges*. Government Office for Science (http://www.bis.gov.uk/assets/foresight/docs/mental-capital/mental_health.pdf).

Rai, D., Skapinakis, P., Wiles, N., *et al* (2010) Common mental disorders, subthreshold symptoms and disability: longitudinal study. *British Journal of Psychiatry*, **197**, 411–412.

Rose, G. (1992) *The Strategy of Preventive Medicine*. Oxford University Press.

van Os, J., Linscott, R. J., Myin-Germeys, I., *et al* (2009) A systematic review and meta-analysis of the psychosis continuum: evidence for a psychosis proneness–persistence–impairment model of psychotic disorder. *Psychological Medicine*, **39**, 179–195.

Wilson, M. (2009) *Delivering Race Equality in Mental Health Care: A Review*. Department of Health (http://www.nmhdu.org.uk/silo/files/delivering-race-equality-in-mental-health-care-a-review.pdf).

CHAPTER 17

Can you do psychotherapy through an interpreter?

Kamaldeep Bhui

The challenges of providing therapies in a culturally and racially diverse society have been reviewed elsewhere (Bhui & Morgan, 2007). In this chapter, I consider the individual psychotherapy frame, which involves two people meeting to discuss the mind of one of them. The encounter involves trust, a human relationship and a sense of connecting with another person in that trusting relationship, so that the client is able to bring their worries, distress, maladies and tragedies into the conversation. The symbolism of the place of healing and the status and power of the healer become relevant as the context of an emotionally charged relationship through which recovery takes place. This notion of therapy presumes that bringing such information into the conversation is culturally sanctioned and seen as a way of improving distress and illness. The client risks rejection and loss of understanding about the personalised meaning of the tragedy; the task involves sharing mental experiences and memories, putting words to them, articulating thoughts about them, questioning these thoughts and the construction of the memories and experiences.

The very act of talking about and putting into words deep personal emotional experience formed from the present and the past results in an alienation of the words from the experience (Nobus, 2000). Communication of internal states of mind is difficult even in a shared language. Across languages and cultures, the task must include slow and paced review of all that is thought to be known and assumed by both therapist and patient. This can undermine any modality of therapy, leading to unexplained drop out from treatment and therefore a lack of effectiveness, what Morgan (1998) has called the 'silence of race'.

Group therapy and family therapy pose specific challenges, as the mental material of many individuals is revealed for its historical interactions, with varying and perhaps contradictory accounts found in the reconstructions of the same events, and all to be discussed, reflected upon, challenged and then worked through emotionally. Such processes will seem as alien to some patients as might rituals to address Jinn or Zar possession are to some therapists. Yet we ask people on entering the consultation and treatment environment to entrust to us their cherished mind and to trust in us not to trample on its precious contents – even more reason why the personal qualities, experiences, background and communication style as well as the profession-specific skills of therapists become important.

Several other chapters in this volume (Chapters 3, 4, 5, 8 and 12) set out the value of involving interpreters and guidance on using a professional interpreter who is present at all sessions with a particular patient. The interpreter should not be seen as a technical translator without a mind, and without transference and countertransference entanglements within the therapeutic relationship. In interpreted therapy, the task of the therapist becomes greater, the professional skills of the interpreter need to be optimal, and the patient has to bear a slowness of pace and progress and more clarifications than would be expected if therapist and patient shared a language and culture. It is such a significant and challenging task, to contain fragments of another's mind and communications and to tenaciously build an image of their internal world, that most therapists will hesitate to take it on through an interpreter. Even if they decide to offer a therapy, most will not begin it with the same expectations of recovery and be able to proceed with the same intensity or depth. If embarked on, the task may later be abandoned without completion. Or it might be heroically pursued, with the potential for success, but also the risk of failure or even greater distress and disappointment for the patient.

Using the same interpreter, with whom pre- and post-therapy sessions are used to calibrate and reflect, can lead to a greater potential for the therapeutic sessions themselves to be less speculative or unclear, especially in relation to psychodynamic meanings, irrespective of the modality of the therapy. I have worked with interpreters in this way in psychosexual clinics, group therapies and individual dynamic and cognitive–behavioural therapies, all moving slowly, with longer assessment phases, with more checking out and clarification, and with careful meaning-making during the therapy. All this needs to be done within the emotionally charged, professionally friendly and containing atmosphere that experienced and trained professionals can create. However, the impingements on this potential therapy are significant, from resources for well-trained inter- preters, restrictions on duration of sessions and treatments, to the inevitable moments when the patient acts out or the therapist enacts an unknown script, all potentially challenging progress towards recovery.

These considerations change my original question from 'Can you do psychotherapy through an interpreter?' to 'Are you prepared to do psychotherapy through an interpreter? Is the interpreter prepared? Is the commissioner prepared? Is the finance director prepared?'.

Some of the practical considerations include knowing the interpreter well, their specific cultural subgroup, language and attitudes to race and culture, their latent identities, and specific details and accompanying contexts of their cultural histories. All of these things can then be factored into the therapist's understanding of material from the patient. This assumes that the therapist has developed the same understanding about their own biography. Historical events, narratives about cultural victories and defeats, about discrimination and about desire and positive feelings of love and affection involving race and culture will impinge on the process. Knowing this about the self, the patient and the interpreter and then working with it creatively, courageously and sensitively are the key tasks for the therapist in interpreted psychotherapy.

References

Bhui, K. & Morgan, N. (2007) Effective psychotherapy in a racially and culturally diverse society. *Advances in Psychiatric Treatment*, **13**, 187–193.

Morgan, H. (1998) Between fear and blindness: the white therapist and the black patient. *Journal of the British Association of Psychotherapists*, **34**, 48–61.

Nobus, D. (2000) *Jacques Lacan and the Freudian Practice of Psychoanalysis*. Routledge.

CHAPTER 18

Can race and racism be acknowledged in the transference without it becoming a source of therapeutic impasse?

Kamaldeep Bhui

Racism has many definitions, some of which identify frank prejudice and verbal or physical hostility towards people with a different racial appearance. Some definitions emphasise the presence of negative and disadvantaging behaviours and attitudes towards the racial other, even among those considering themselves liberal and taking an anti-racist stance (Bhui, 2002; Primm, 2006). It is well established that, as a scientific construct, race does not determine how likely a person is to get a mental illness, and it does not really predict social, cultural or ethnic characteristics. Its importance lies mainly in the propensity for human populations to make use of a shorthand to describe and attempt to classify each other (often incorrectly) on the basis of appearance. It is also important because power, income and status appear to be patterned by race.

Given that in therapeutic settings, patient and therapist have many expectations of each other, race becomes one of numerous characteristics that both make use of in their initial encounter. Then it is taken up in the life of the consultation, assessment and treatment cycle, or it remains very silent, as if nothing to do with either person. This observation has been repeatedly made by clinicians and therapists for many decades. It has become known as the 'silence of race', carrying with it a quality of the repression or disavowal of an experience or set of historical group relations that would otherwise be troublesome (Young-Bruehl, 1998; Qureshi, 2007). When race does arise in a more explicit manner, it is difficult for therapist and patient to know how to take it up, given that it might lead to very different and deep-seated responses from either. When it is mentioned, it can be lightly touched upon and then overlooked or laughed off, perhaps disguising contempt or disgust, or shame or guilt, or some of those automatic thoughts and feelings that emerge in relationships. Fantasies of miscegenation, for example, are common (Calvo, 2008) in cross-racial encounters, and are often found at times of war and conflict, when inter-group (race, tribe, nation) relationships are attacked. If deeper feelings about race are permitted to emerge or erupt, something that the therapist will be sensitive to, this need not mean the end of the therapeutic alliance or relationship. Rather, it is perhaps an opportunity to deepen it. However, many – if not most – analysts and therapists feel that race is a taboo area, much like religion, that tends not to be considered much in professional training, personal analyses or postgraduate curricula. They therefore may not feel equipped to work with it.

Understanding comments related to race when they emerge, and their transferential implications, is as important as understanding counter-transferential responses related to or grounded in the race of the patient and the professional, even if this is perplexing and difficult to manage for patient and therapist. In one sense the fragility, fear, concern, terror and, at the same time, curiosity and interest in the racial other and racial references, are understandable given that the phenotype of racism most commonly known about is the more frank prejudicial variety, perhaps associated with international conflict, atrocity, homicide, torture or mutilation. National and local media reflect collective myths and symbols that perhaps reflect this better-known phenotype. Nobody wishes to be identified with it or to be a victim of it, so the task to apprehend material with racial and racism-related content is challenging; but it need not be seen as a totally different class of expression or experience, without a useful message of therapeutic or anti-therapeutic significance.

Hamer (2006) talks of racism as a regressed state of transference, characterised by polarised representations of self and other, categorical thinking, and the predominance of splitting and projection as defences. The racial transference can express hostility, hatred, fear, powerlessness and all that goes with the history of Black–White relations as represented in the unconscious (Dalal, 2006). The patient should be permitted to express such views without fear of catastrophe. Indeed, such emotions may be present so subtly that effort needs to be expended to notice them and subject them to scrutiny so that they can be better understood. Otherwise, important aspects of the therapeutic relationship will sink away into silence. So race talk may come to serve as a vehicle for the expression of the negative transference. It may offer a way for people to share the pain of abusive experiences, of isolation, discrimination, of lost lands and identities, or just differences that can be explored.

The demands of such work are high for both therapist and patient. It can be exhausting, upsetting, wounding and traumatic. It can assault cherished identities or sacred historical markers and events that are a core part of personal identity. Therefore, this work is not easily recommended in routine practice and it should be undertaken only with sufficiently experienced and informed therapists and supervisors who have the ability and capacity to explore these powerful fantasies, images, identities and the related impulses and shifts in states of mind that accompany trauma.

Listening out for and hearing one's own reactions and internal dialogue in response to the patient's talk about race and racism is a helpful way of permitting material to emerge. Intervention should wait until more is understood and the therapeutic relationship is well established. The therapeutic alliance is critical to the working through of a strong negative transference, especially if it arises early in therapy. It is also critical to the avoidance of superficial therapeutic work based on accepting narratives of transference that have not been investigated or explored. Gelso & Mohr (2001) discuss at length the many definitions of transference and countertransference, and the necessity of understanding these in order to deepen the therapeutic alliance. Conversely, an alliance is itself necessary to the working through of the transference and countertransference, both of which are co-created, a product of the internal worlds of patient and therapist. Importantly, the therapist must be sure that it is safe to begin working through the transference and countertransference within the therapy. Introducing the term 'racial/ethnic or sexual orientation minority' (RSM) status, Gelso & Mohr suggest that different RSM pairings of therapist and patient result in different ways in which the working alliance, transference and countertransference unfold.

Helms & Cook (1999) anticipate that some of the cultural transference symbolises past traumatic experiences that the patient (or his or her identity group) encountered with the therapist's identity group. Experiences and fears of oppression become manifest through the status difference between patient and therapist. Some of the patient's experiences and perceptions are grounded in reality, and should be recognised as such. The task of the therapist is to disentangle the transferential meaning given to real experiences from the experiences themselves, so that the patient's reality is not dismissed. Dismissing the patient's reality is a risk, as the negative transference may recreate the negative feelings in the therapist that the patient anticipates in a cross-racial, cross-ethnic or cross-cultural group pairing. However, a therapist of the same racial, ethnic or cultural group as the patient is also not without risk, as an early positive working alliance may give way to transference expectations of accommodation and to idealisation, which if not met are felt even more deeply as failures. Gelso & Mohr (2001) assert that these issues are endemic to therapies and need not cause therapeutic impasse or failure. Understanding racism and racial transference at this deeper level and acknowledging splits in the ego permits the rational, reasonable and observing self to deepen the working alliance irrespective of emotional impulses and eruptions.

References

Bhui, K. (ed.) (2002) *Racism & Mental Health: Prejudice and Suffering*. Jessica Kingsley
Calvo, L. (2008) Racial fantasies and the primal scene of miscegenation. *International Journal of Psychoanalysis*, **89**, 55–70.

Dalal, F. (2006) Racism: processes of detachment, dehumanization, and hatred. *Psychoanalytic Quarterly*, **75**, 131–161.

Gelso, C. J. & Mohr, J. J. (2001) The working alliance and the transference/counter-transference relationship: their manifestation with racial/ethnic and sexual orientation minority clients and therapists. *Applied and Preventive Psychology*, **10**, 51–68.

Hamer, F. M. (2006) Racism as a transference state: episodes of racial hostility in the psychoanalytic context. *Psychoanalytic Quarterly*, **75**, 197–214.

Helms, J. E. & Cook, D. A. (1999) *Using Race and Culture in Counselling and Psychotherapy: Theory and Process*. Allyn & Bacon.

Primm, A. B. (2006) Understanding the significance of race in the psychiatric clinical setting. *Focus*, **4**, 6–8.

Qureshi, A. (2007) I was being myself but being an actor too: the experience of a Black male in interracial psychotherapy. *Psychology and Psychotherapy: Theory, Research and Practice*, **80**, 467–479.

Young-Bruehl, E. (1998) *The Anatomy of Prejudice*. Harvard University Press.

CHAPTER 19

Cultural competence: models, measures and movements

Kamaldeep Bhui

A few years ago, colleagues and I undertook a systematic review of the literature on cultural competence in mental healthcare (Bhui *et al*, 2007). This revealed many interpretations of the concept, from which we synthesised a composite definition of cultural competence as the set of skills and processes that enable mental health professionals to provide services that are culturally appropriate for the diverse populations that they serve. This set focused on professionally defined outcomes, and included attention to obvious language differences in the consultation, as well as to how culture influences attitudes, expressions of distress and help-seeking practices. Showing respect for the patient's cultural beliefs and attitudes was an important component, especially when their views opposed or differed from those of the professional. Emphasis was given to a genuine willingness and desire to learn about other cultures, rather than seeing such learning as a managerial requirement or an imposition. There is some hostility towards the notion of cultural competence, which suggests the belief that there is nothing more to be learnt. It might be thought that all psychiatrists should already possess the necessary skills, but we know that this is not the case. Many admit to needing help, courses and accreditation, and, were the skills and aptitudes already there, books such as this would be neither necessary nor attractive (Bennett *et al*, 2007).

The definitions indicate a common aim, to improve performance and increase the capabilities of staff providing services for people from ethnic minorities. A popular definition from the National Center for Cultural Competence (2006) in the USA reads:

'Cultural competence requires that organizations:

- have a defined set of values and principles, and demonstrate behaviors, attitudes, policies and structures that enable them to work effectively cross-culturally.
- have the capacity to (1) value diversity, (2) conduct self-assessment, (3) manage the dynamics of difference, (4) acquire and institutionalize cultural knowledge and (5) adapt to diversity and the cultural contexts of the communities they serve.
- incorporate the above in all aspects of policy making, administration, practice, service delivery and involve systematically consumers, key stakeholders and communities.'

However, other brands of cultural competence have emerged (Bhui *et al*, 2012). Race equality and cultural capability (RECC) training (Box 19.1) arose from the Department of Health's Delivering Race Equality in Mental Health programme. As part of the programme, a survey was conducted of the range and types of race equality training provided by mental health services in England (Bennett *et al*, 2007). The findings of this survey are summarised in Box 19.2. A cultural consultation service offers one way of achieving the objectives set out in Box 19.2. One such service has been set up in Canada to collaborate with existing services in mental health, psychiatry and primary care (Kirmayer *et al*, 2003). Mental health practitioners and primary care clinicians refer patients (or their case files) to the service for a cultural consultation based on an expanded version of the DSM-IV cultural formulation and making use of cultural consultants and culture brokers. Kirmayer *et al*'s evaluation of the service revealed that clinicians on the whole welcomed this sort of intervention and that in many cases it led to changes in the clinical management plans for individual patients.

This volume is a contribution to workforce development and the cultural competence of psychiatrists and others working in mental health specialties. However, the assumption that cultural competence is simply an educational intervention underestimates the task (Bhui *et al*, 2012). Many other factors must be considered: the personal biographies of individual professionals; the meaning and salience for them of cultural and racial identities; their levels of curiosity to learn about other people; and their willingness to acknowledge diversity, to not assume that all people require systematically delivered universal interventions and to accept that they might need to learn additional skills that encourage empathy and understanding and

---

Box 19.1   Race equality and cultural capability (RECC)

The principles and values of the RECC programme are given as:

1   Dealing with inequality and not just cultural difference
2   Having a deeper understanding of culture
3   RECC is an ordinary part of good practice
4   Services will improve only through a 'whole systems' approach
5   Greater BME service user participation leads to greater appropriateness of services
6   Miscommunication often leads to unnecessary conflicts
7   We need to recognise institutional discrimination as a problem before we can begin to tackle it properly
8   Know yourself first before trying to understand others
9   Unacknowledged prejudices grow in power and influence
10 Values are central to mental health practice

(Fern Associates, 2006)

Box 19.2   Results and conclusions of the Sainsbury Centre for Mental Health's review of cultural competency training in England

Training objectives and content

84% of employees and 91% of providers said one of the main aims of training was to improve awareness of race and cultural issues. 80% of training providers but only 33% of staff thought changing behaviour was among the key aims.

The content of training varied widely. It was influenced most by the trainer's own perspectives and the commissioning organisation's requirements.

The most common reported contents were policy and legal issues (88%) and understanding difference (82%). Less common contents included skills for non-discriminatory practice (60%) and strategies for resolving conflict (39%).

One quarter of participants reported that service users were involved in delivering the training.

Training providers

There is no professional body that sets standards for the qualifications and practice of race related training providers. 60% of training providers in our survey had received training in race equality, 54% in mental health care and 40% in training skills.

45% of trainers were independent or freelance providers. 34% reported that they use or have used mental health services.

Evaluation of training

35% of statutory and half of independent sector organisations had evaluated the training their staff received. The main methods of evaluation were attendance at training events (76%) and post-training reaction (71%).

One-third of commissioners said training had had a positive impact.

77% of training participants in our survey reported some positive impact on their work or themselves, but only 48% reported a positive impact on the organisation or service delivery.

Conclusions and recommendations

This report concludes that:

- Current approaches to race equality training are inappropriate and inadequate in addressing racial inequality in mental health services.
- Essentially 'training for race equality' should focus specifically on the areas of inequality people experience in mental health services, such as diagnosis, compulsory detention, reducing fear etc., rather than a generic focus on cultural difference or diversity.
- Emphasis in race related training must be on the improvement of professional practice and not merely the acquisition of knowledge on the cultures of those categorised as the 'other'.
- Training for race equality should form part of a wider framework for reducing race inequality, embedded within the organisation's clinical governance systems. It should address the needs of the organisation and its staff and form part of a wider framework of reducing race inequality

(Reproduced with permission from Bennett *et al*, 2007: pp. 7–8)

engagement. Some see the emphasis on race as excessive or that on culture as defensive and avoidant of the core inequalities that are so apparent in mental healthcare. Engaging with the discourse requires that all manage the entanglements that arise, and requires significant understanding of the power of cultural, racial, ethnic and religious symbols and identities in the minds of both patients and professionals.

Furthermore, alongside this essential requirement for professionals, reflecting aptitude and attitudes, is an ever-expanding knowledge base about social, pharmacological and psychological interventions and their adaptation and effectiveness in culturally and racially diverse groups.

We do need generic measures of cultural competence in the workforce. Developing outcome measures of cultural competency is difficult. One small randomised trial showed that the type of teaching (lecture *v.* experiential; epidemiological *v.* anthropological approach) influenced the way medical students responded to a case vignette: those who had received experiential teaching using a more anthropological approach proposed more psychosocial interventions than those who had received standard lecture-based teaching (Chakraborty *et al*, 2009). The American Academy of Medical Colleges has produced a measure of curriculum quality with regard to the teaching of cultural competence (Lie *et al*, 2006). The website of the London Deanery serving National Health Service doctors and dentists gives much information on cultural competence, including definitions, resources and tools, and suitable courses for postgraduate study (http://www.londondeanery.ac.uk/var/equality-diversity/cultural-competence).

References

Bennett, J., Kalathil, J. & Keating, F. (2007) *Race Equality Training in Mental Health Services in England: Does One Size Fit All?* Sainsbury Centre for Mental Health.

Bhui, K., Warfa, N., Edonya, P., *et al* (2007) Cultural competence in mental health care: a review of model evaluations. *BMC Health Services Research*, **31** (7), 15.

Bhui, K., Ascoli, M. & Nuamh, O. (2012) The place of race and racism in cultural competence: what can we learn from the English experience about the narratives of evidence and argument? *Transcultural Psychiatry*, **49**, 185–205.

Chakraborty, A., McKenzie, K., Bhui, K., *et al* (2009) A randomised control trial (RCT) of undergraduate cross-cultural psychiatry training. *World Cultural Psychiatry Research Review*, **4**, 63–73.

Fern Associates (2006) *Introduction to RECC Training*. Fern Associates (http://www.fernsassociates.co.uk/site/view/RECCdownloads).

Kirmayer, L. J., Groleau, D., Guzder, J., *et al* (2003) Cultural consultation: a model for mental health services for multicultural societies. *Canadian Journal of Psychiatry*, **48**, 145–153.

Lie, D., Boker, J. & Cleveland, E. (2006) Using the tool for assessing cultural competence training (TACCT) to measure faculty and medical student perceptions of cultural competence instruction in the first three years of the curriculum. *Academic Medicine*, **81**, 557–564.

National Center for Cultural Competence (2006) *Conceptual Frameworks/Models, Guiding Values and Principles*. Georgetown University Center for Child and Human Development (http://www11.georgetown.edu/research/gucchd/nccc/foundations/frameworks.html).

CHAPTER 20

Religion, spirituality and mental health

Imran Ali

The past decade has seen a surge of interest among health professionals in the integration of religious and spiritual matters into mental healthcare. However, this forgotten dimension has played a significant role in many people's lives for centuries. It may come as a surprise to find that the first psychiatric hospitals were built in Baghdad in 705 AD, and in Cairo in 800 AD (Youssef & Youssef, 1996). Religious therapy was an integral part of treatment in these early institutions.

Many authors offer definitions of the concept of spirituality in relation to healthcare. These include having a sense of purpose, searching for peace, understanding the world, and engaging in practices that give meaning to individual lives. However, one needs to define spirituality with care in order not to narrow its meaning too far: any definition should reflect spirituality's importance in giving meaning to experiences (Rumbold, 2007) and be inclusive of diverse religious views (Canda & Furman, 2010).

A potential shortcoming of existing practice is the use of generic spiritual assessment tools without considering the underlying assumptions inherent in the healthcare systems for which they are developed (Rumbold, 2007). Many hospitals have developed resource files listing religious and spiritual rituals and 'dos and don'ts', but these often overlook the deeper meanings behind people's religious beliefs and attitudes and how these affect their mental health and well-being.

Many people with mental health problems want their spiritual needs to be addressed, but often lack confidence in nursing staff and fear being misunderstood (Koslander & Arvidsson, 2007). In a US survey of 1413 patients visiting family practices, of the 921 respondents, 83% wanted physicians to ask about their spiritual beliefs under certain circumstances (McGord et al, 2004). Spirituality offers moments of reflection, opportunity to search for change; without these moments something is missing (Dadich, 2007). Spiritual beliefs can play a positive role in mental health and suicide prevention (Coghlan & Ali, 2009). Incorporating spirituality in the care of people with schizophrenia can promote coping strategies and help with recovery (Mohr & Huguelet, 2004). Religious beliefs and practices are commonly used to help people cope with mental distress.

A study of coping styles in six ethnic groups found that 'religious coping' (which included prayer, using amulets and trust in God) was common and promoted resilience and recovery (Bhui *et al*, 2008).

How well are religion and spirituality integrated into cross-cultural research? Tarakeshwar *et al* (2003) reviewed the contents of four major cross-cultural psychology journals over the previous 34 years. Only 2–6% of studies considered religious variables. Of the research that does consider spirituality in mental health, most is quantitative in method, is focused at Judaism and Christianity, and relies on Christian terminology in the survey questions (Cornah, 2006).

There is much to learn from religious practices that have been prevalent for centuries and have helped countless people in their life journey. Hinduism is one of the oldest religions. Ancient Indian Ayurvedic texts describe mental illness, ascribing madness to disregard of God or inadequate diet, and other psychiatric symptoms to imbalance of bodily fluids (Bhugra, 1996). Modern Ayurvedic therapy includes offerings to *Agni* (fire), one of the five elements thought to compose the universe and the human body, and the use of talismans and charms (Bhugra, 1992). These practices may be used in conjunction with medication and consultations with doctors. Patients may also be encouraged to worship in the temple as part of their treatment (Somasundaram, 1973).

Spiritual healing is an essential component in Muslim traditions. The concepts of *qalb* (heart), *nafs* (spirit), *ruh* (soul) and *aql* (intellect) are key principles. Abu Zayd Al-Balkhi, a famous Muslim physician and polymath of the 10th century AD criticised practitioners who concentrated only on the physical aspects of health and emphasised the holistic treatment of both body and soul (Badri, 1998). The heart, rather than the mind, is seen as the seat of intellectual function. Spiritual diseases of the heart are divided into two categories: *Shubuhat*, or obfuscations, which impair understanding; and *Shahawat*, which are linked with urges or desires.

In Sikhism, people avoid five passions which are seen as obstacles along their spiritual path. These are *kam* (lust), *lobh* (greed), *krodh* (rage), *moh* (attachment) and *ahankar* (ego or pride). Death and loss are dealt with through the concepts of a life cycle in which the individual returns in another form.

What are the implications for clinical practice?

Taking a spiritual history can capture important experiences and perceptions. There is some disagreement as to whose responsibility it is to assess spiritual care. The role of the physician may be to ensure that spirituality has been assessed and to involve specialists such as imams, rabbis and clergymen in more thorough assessments and treatment (Handzo & Koenig, 2004). D'Souza & George (2006) argue that all medical students and graduates should be trained in taking a spiritual history. Cox (1996) echoes a similar opinion: taking a religious history with any linked spiritual meanings should be a routine part of a psychiatric assessment. Respect and acknowledgement of the significance of religious beliefs and spirituality in people's lives is important.

Koenig (2008) has suggested praying with the patient if they ask for this, but there is a view this may blur professional boundaries (Poole *et al*, 2008).

How do spirituality and religion relate to each other? Are they one and the same or interconnected, or are these two totally separate things? Each patient may vary in their understanding of these concepts, as much as professionals may vary, so a good practice point is to ask rather than assume what is the case for each person. For Muslims, spirituality equates to *Ihsan*, which means achieving excellence, and this is done through strengthening their relationships with God, with themselves and with God's creation. *Ihsan* is not seen in isolation but alongside *Iman* (referring to inward actions) and *Islam* (referring to outward actions). Some professionals do not feel comfortable asking about or even using the term religion. In a survey of 231 consultants and trainees working in London teaching hospitals, 27% reported a religious affiliation and 23% believed in God (Neeleman & King, 1993). In such cases, the word spirituality is used as a catch-all phrase to encompass both religion and spirituality, and this may disguise a religious or spiritual dissonance between professionals and patients. One study in the UK found that patients' religious beliefs were ignored unless they were associated with psychopathology (Hilton *et al*, 2002). An experienced practitioner is mindful of not imposing their own views onto others, but this may still be a concern in relation to religion and spiritual beliefs. Do professionals and patients feel comfortable discussing spiritual issues in a largely secular society? The inclusion of religious practitioners such as imams, rabbis and vicars in the multidisciplinary team may provide further insight in both assessment and treatment.

How should psychological therapies be modified for people from Black and minority ethnic groups, who may have different religious needs than the majority population in the UK? One can fall into a self-deception that translating material and conducting therapy sessions in the patient's native language is sufficient. It is not. The case formulation itself needs to be deeper, taking into consideration religious, spiritual and cultural dimensions of illness and of care. Listening and learning from patients' spiritual experiences and from religious and spiritual practices that have survived centuries can open a door onto a new dimension in mental healthcare, one that we have only just begun to explore.

References

Badri, M. B. (1998) Abu-Zayd Al-Balkhi: a genius whose psychiatric contributions needed more than ten centuries to be appreciated. *Malaysian Journal of Psychiatry*, **6**, 1–6.

Bhugra, D. (1992) Psychiatry in ancient Indian texts: a review. *History of Psychiatry*, **3**, 167–186.

Bhugra, D. (1996) Hinduism and Ayurveda. In *Psychiatry and Religion: Context, Consensus and Controversies* (ed. D. Bhugra), pp. 97–111. Routledge.

Bhui, K., King, M., Dein, S., *et al* (2008) Ethnicity and religious coping with mental distress. *Journal of Mental Health*, **17**, 141–151.

Canda, E. R. & Furman, L. E. (2010) *Spiritual Diversity in Social Work Practice: The Heart of Helping* (2nd edn). Oxford University Press.

Coghlan C. & Ali, I. (2009) Suicide. In *Spirituality and Psychiatry* (eds C. Cook, A. Powell & A. Sims), pp. 61–80. RCPsych Publications.

Cornah, D. (2006) *The Impact of Spirituality on Mental Health: A Review of the Literature.* Mental Health Foundation.

Cox, J. L. (1996) Psychiatry and religion: a general psychiatrist's perspective. In *Psychiatry and Religion: Context, Consensus and Controversies* (ed. D. Bhugra), pp. 157–166. Routledge.

Dadich, A. (2007) Is spirituality important to young people in recovery? Insights from participants of self-help support groups. *Southern Medical Journal*, **100**, 422–425.

D'Souza, R. & George, K. (2006) Spirituality, religion and psychiatry: its application to clinical practice. *Australasian Psychiatry*, **14**, 408–412.

Handzo, G. & Koenig, H. (2004) Spiritual care: whose job is it anyway? *Southern Medical Journal*, **97**, 1242–1244.

Hilton, C., Ghaznavi, F. & Zuberi, T. (2002) Religious beliefs and practices in acute mental health patients. *Nursing Standard*, **51**, 33–36.

Koenig, H. G. (2008) Religion and mental health: what should psychiatrists do? *Psychiatric Bulletin*, **32**, 201–203.

Koslander, T. & Arvidsson, B. (2005) How the spiritual dimension is addressed in psychiatric patient–nurse relationships. *Journal of Advanced Nursing*, **51**, 558–566.

Koslander, T. & Arvidsson, B. (2007) Patients' conceptions of how spiritual dimension is addressed in the psychiatric patient–nurse relationship: a qualitative study. *Journal of Advanced Nursing*, **57**, 597–604.

McGord, G., Gilchrist, V. J., Grossman, S. D., *et al* (2004) Discussing spirituality with patients: a rational and ethical approach. *Annals of Family Medicine*, **2**, 356–361.

Mohr, S. & Huguelet, P. (2004) The relationship between schizophrenia and religion and its implications for care. *Swiss Medical Weekly*, **134**, 369–376.

Neeleman, J. & King, M. B. (1993) Psychiatrist's religious attitudes in relation to their clinical practice: a survey of 231 psychiatrists. *Acta Psychiatrica Scandinavica*, **88**, 420–424.

Poole, R., Higgo, R., Strong, G., *et al* (2008) Religion, psychiatry and professional boundaries. *Psychiatric Bulletin*, **32**, 356–357.

Rumbold, B. D. (2007) A review of spiritual assessment in health care practice. *Medical Journal of Australia*, **186** (suppl. 10), S60–S62.

Somasundaram, O. (1973) Religious treatment of mental illness in Tamil Nadu. *Indian Journal of Psychiatry*, **15**, 38–48.

Tarakeshwar, N., Stanton, J. & Pargament, K. I. (2003) Religion: an overlooked dimension in cross-cultural psychology. *Journal of Cross-Cultural Psychology*, **34**, 377–394.

Youssef, H. A. & Youssef, F. A. (1996) Evidence for the existence of schizophrenia in medieval Islamic society. *History of Psychiatry*, **7**, 55–62.

Index

Compiled by Linda English

Page numbers in *italics* refer to figures or boxes